SELF-CARE ESSENTIALS

A SIMPLE GUIDE TO MANAGING YOUR HEALTH CARE AND LIVING WELL

Copyright and Disclosure

Self-Care Essentials: A Simple Guide to Managing Your Health Care and Living Well

EXECUTIVE EDITOR
David M. Hunnicutt, Ph.D.
President, Wellness Councils of America

AUTHORS
Chad Abresch, M.Ed., Craig Johnson, and Bo Abresch
Wellness Councils of America

DESIGNER
Paul Burner, Slide Arts Graphic Design
www.slidearts.com

PUBLISHED AND DISTRIBUTED BY
The Wellness Councils of America (WELCOA)
9802 Nicholas Street, Suite 315
Omaha, NE 68114-2106

Phone: (402) 827-3590
Fax: (402) 827-3594

WEBSITE: www.welcoa.org
E-MAIL: wellworkplace@welcoa.org

© 2001 Wellness Councils of America

Table of Contents

ESSENTIAL...
Acknowledgements

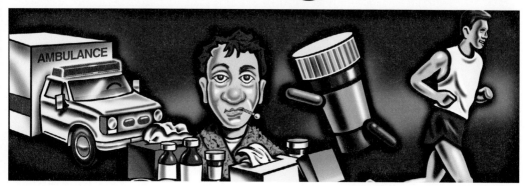

Dear Reader,

This premiere edition of Self-Care Essentials has been carefully researched and written in a manner that is easy to understand and apply to everyday living. We trust that you, the reader, will be able to take away critical information that can safeguard health, treat illness, and improve well-being for yourself and your loved ones.

Self-Care Essentials would not be possible without the expert advice and guidance of many health professionals. Their years of scholarship, work in the field, and willingness to make this book a reality are greatly appreciated.

We are deeply indebted to the following people:

Christina M. Hunnicutt, Ph.D.

Thomas C. Howard, M.D.

Karen J. Stacey, M.D.

We would also like to give special attention and thanks to Dr. David Chenoweth for his consultation and review of materials.

David Hunnicutt, Ph.D.

President

Healthy Essentials

Self-Care Essentials is a simple guide to managing your health care and living well. In this age of medical advancement, knowing how to best care for your health and the health of your family can be a tricky business. That's why reliable and easy-to-understand health information is a must. And that's exactly what this book offers. Here's what you'll find in the following pages.

CHAPTER ONE: EMERGENCY CARE

Whether it's a minor scrape or a life-threatening head injury, you'll know what to do and when to call for help in an emergency situation.

CHAPTER TWO: OUR MOST COMMON CONDITIONS

In this chapter, we'll cover 28 of the most common medical conditions grouped into 12 categories. The information will provide legitimate solutions that you can implement at home.

CHAPTER THREE: CHRONIC CONDITIONS

Even if you suffer from a chronic condition, effective treatment strategies are available. This chapter will key in on those strategies and provide a means for better living.

CHAPTER FOUR: TAKING MEDICATIONS

Medications are a valuable weapon in the self-care arsenal. In this chapter, we'll provide critical information for getting the most out of medications.

GLOSSARY

In this valuable section, you'll find 100 plus definitions of medical terms and conditions that will help guide your efforts to care for your health and well-being.

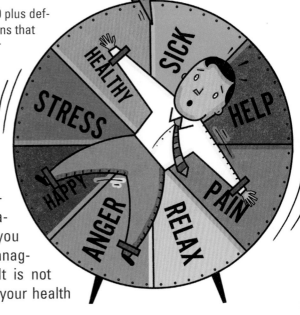

...Before we dive into the details, let's first look at some information that is critical to healthy living. We encourage you to learn the following healthy essentials and do your best to live by them. Also, it's important to understand that the information provided here is to help you become better informed about managing your health and living well. It is not intended to replace the advice of your health care provider.

Physical Activity

Physical activity is not an all-or-nothing affair. Even if it's just a short walk after dinner, physical activity is a must.

How much physical activity is enough?

■ The Surgeon General recommends a moderate amount of physical activity on most, if not all days of the week—here's just some of what you can do:

 ✓ 30 minutes of brisk walking or raking leaves

 ✓ 15 minutes of running

 ✓ 45 minutes of playing volleyball

 ✓ Greater amounts of physical activity are encouraged if time and health conditions allow

When is the best time to exercise?

■ Physical activity is beneficial at most any time of day (to help ensure a good night's rest, it is best to avoid intense exercise 4 hours before bedtime)

■ Try to schedule your workouts at the same time every day—make exercise a priority and part of your daily routine

What types of exercise should I be doing?

■ It is best to include both cardiovascular exercise and strength training in your workouts

■ Cardiovascular exercises increase your heart rate and improve your ability to use oxygen—here's just some of what you can do:
 ✓ Walking   ✓ Running   ✓ Hiking
 ✓ Swimming   ✓ Bicycling

■ Strength training is primarily aimed at increasing the tone, strength, and/or size of your muscles and is performed by moving your body against resistance, as with weight lifting

WORDS TO THE WISE

Together, physical activity and nutrition largely determine weight. This is why the best way to control weight is to let weight control itself by getting enough physical activity and eating right.

ESSENTIAL TIPS ON...

Nutrition

The information surrounding proper nutrition can seem a little confusing, even contradictory at times. The truth, however, is that good nutrition can be fairly simple.

Calories count

- Simply put, if you consume more calories than you use, you'll gain weight
- On the other hand, if you consume fewer calories than you use, you'll lose weight
- To lose weight, adjust your total number of daily calories down slowly (any extra pounds should come off the same way they went on—little by little)

Variety matters

- Here's how much the experts recommend we eat per day from each of the food groups:
  ✓ Bread, cereal, rice, and pasta—6 to 11 servings
  ✓ Vegetables—3 to 5 servings
  ✓ Fruits—2 to 4 servings
  ✓ Milk, yogurt, and cheese—2 to 3 servings
  ✓ Meat, poultry, fish, dry beans, eggs, and nuts—2 to 3 servings
  ✓ Fats, oils, and sweets—use these foods sparingly

Balance is everything

- Diets that recommend eating only one food or from only one food group are not healthy
- The key to a healthy diet is a limited number of daily calories with the proper balance of servings from each of the food groups

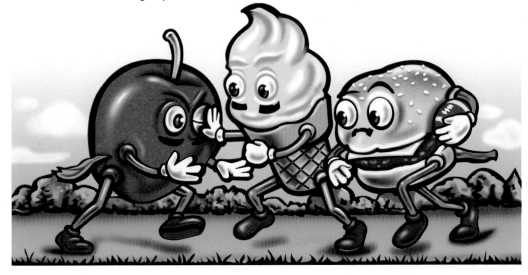

ESSENTIAL TIPS ON...

Stress

When it comes to maintaining good health, keeping stress at bay is key. Stress is an attack on the body that compromises our defense system. Controlling stress can be tough in our fast-paced lives, but not impossible. A few key tricks can be extremely helpful.

Broaden your perspective

■ Try to think about upcoming events with anticipation rather than anxiety

■ Remember that current discomforts are rarely permanent—things change

■ Realize that not all of the aspects of your life or day are stressful

Breathe deeply

■ When you find yourself stressed, try to breathe deeply and just slow down

■ Breathe deeply with your thoughts as well— slow down and control your thoughts

Focus on others

■ Stress is often a result of self-focus—consider others and what you could do to brighten their days

■ Try focusing on kindness toward others when the stress of life mounts

 WORDS TO THE WISE

Some amount of stress is inevitable. In fact, most of us would find a totally stress-free life a bit dull. The key is balance. If stress is something you wrestle with, figure out what factors cause it, and make sure your reaction to those events is reasonable.

ESSENTIAL TIPS ON...

Rest

On average, adults sleep 6 hours and 54 minutes a night during the workweek—more than an hour less than the recommended amount. The answer to our sleep deficit is not as difficult as we tend to make it. Here are some simple tips that can help.

Environment is everything

■ Your bedroom should be conducive to sleep—here's what you can do:

✓ Keep the television out of the bedroom

✓ Make sure your room has plenty of air circulation

✓ Keep the temperature of your room at a moderate level

✓ Some background noise like a fan can be helpful—but be careful, a noisemaker can become addictive

✓ Above all else, set up a bedtime routine—make sleep a habit

Alcohol, caffeine, and tobacco... oh my!

■ Contrary to popular belief, a "nightcap" does not lead to better rest

■ Caffeine should be avoided for 4 hours before going to bed

■ Cigarettes are never a good idea and reduce the quality and quantity of sleep

The other healthy essentials

■ Regular physical activity will improve your quality of sleep

■ Proper nutrition will also improve the quality of your sleep

■ Reducing stress can eliminate insomnia and improve the quality of your sleep

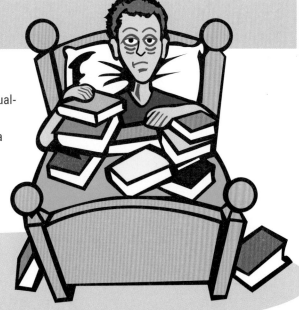

ESSENTIAL TIPS ON...

Preparing for a Doctor's Visit

Self-care treatment alone is sometimes not enough for certain health conditions. In these cases, you may need to see a doctor. By being properly prepared for your visit, you can be sure to get the most out of it and leave with confidence. Here's how to prepare.

Before your visit

- Educate yourself as much as possible on your condition
- Record your exact symptoms, when they occurred, how long they lasted, and what you did to feel better

During your visit

- Tell the doctor what triggered/triggers the condition
- Ask the doctor as many questions as appropriate, such as:
  - ✓ What should I do if new symptoms develop?
  - ✓ When can I expect to feel better?
  - ✓ Are there lifestyle changes I can make to prevent this problem from recurring?
  - ✓ Who should I contact if I have questions?
  - ✓ How and when should I take medications?
  - ✓ Where can I get more information about my condition?

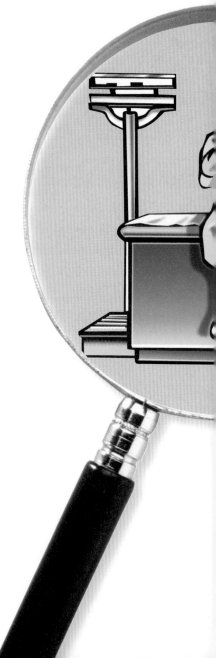

After your visit

- Write down the main points of the visit
- If you received a prescription, ask the pharmacist for detailed information on the medication
- If you think of additional questions, don't hesitate to call the doctor's office and ask
- Tell a family member or friend how the visit went, what the treatment plan is, and when you can expect to feel better

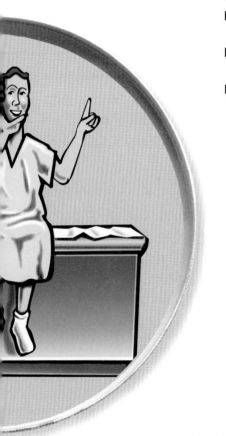

"When I told my doctor I couldn't afford an operation, he offered to touch up my x-rays."

–HENNY YOUNGMAN

WORDS TO THE WISE

Times have changed. Years ago, it seemed we all had a personal physician that knew us and our medical history. Today, this kind of personal medical service is a rarity. The good news is that this doesn't have to affect the quality of our health care. In fact, today we can expect to receive even better health care than in years past. However, we do have to take more personal responsibility. And, preparing for a doctor's visit is an essential part of this responsibility.

ESSENTIAL...

First Aid Equipment

Try as we might to improve safety and live well, accidents can and do happen. A fundamental aspect of being prepared for these accidents is having the essential equipment.

Keep the following items in your first aid kit

Essential medical gear

- Bandages and gauze pads in assorted sizes
- Adhesive medical tape and wound closure tapes
- Elastic wrap
- Syrup of ipecac and activated charcoal
- Acetaminophen, ibuprofen, and aspirin
- Hydrogen peroxide
- Chemical cold packs
- Antibiotic cream, lotion, or spray
- Hydrocortisone cream
- Thermometer and petroleum jelly

Essential odds and ends

- Scissors and tweezers
- Safety pins
- Disposable rubber or latex gloves
- Flashlight
- Emergency phone numbers, including your doctor, hospital, Poison Control Center, fire department, and police station

WORDS TO THE WISE

Having a well-stocked first aid kit will do us no good if we don't have it with us when an emergency strikes. For this reason, you may want to consider investing in a couple of first aid kits. You can keep one in your home and a second in your car in case of a roadside emergency. Check your kit twice a year to avoid damaged or outdated supplies.

WHY...
Self-Care?

Medical self-care is a powerful health information tool. For everyone willing to use it, self-care can improve health and raise quality of life. That's precisely why Self-Care Essentials was written. Take just a moment to review the following questions.

Who is this book for?

- Employees and employers
- The healthy and those in need
- Singles and families
- Teachers and students
- Management teams
- The young and old alike
- In short, it's for anyone who cares about personal health and well-being

What is self-care all about?

- Staying informed
- Educating ourselves and others
- Providing a higher level of personal care
- Peace of mind
- Protection and prevention
- Reducing unnecessary hospital visits and saving money
- Living longer and well

When is self-care appropriate?

- When you have a chronic condition
- In an emergency situation
- When you have questions about medications
- When you want information on specific conditions
- When suffering from day-to-day aches and pains

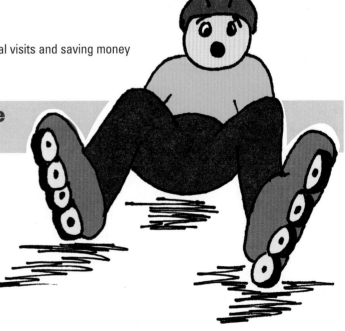

Continued on next page...

WHY...
Self-Care?

Where can self-care be used?

■ In the home
■ At the worksite
■ On the road
■ In schools
■ Outdoors
■ At the gym
■ Anywhere a health-related condition arises

Why Self-Care Essentials?

■ It addresses what to do in emergency situations
■ It informs us about our most common conditions
■ It provides up to date information on chronic conditions
■ It gives valuable information on taking medications
■ It serves as an educational piece on important health issues
■ It can save money on medical costs!

How do I use this book?

■ Keep it in your desk at work
■ Hang it on your refrigerator at home
■ Store it near your medicine cabinet
■ Toss it in the glove box before a road trip
■ Look up a condition when someone gets hurt
■ Bookmark and dog-ear the pages
■ Make notes in the margins
■ Study the sections that
  concern you the most

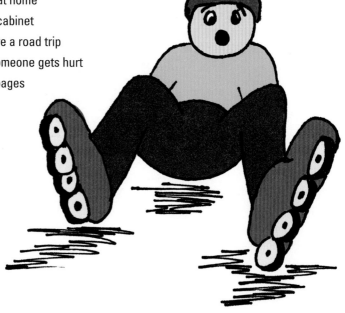

CHAPTER ONE:

Emergency Care

In this chapter of Self-Care Essentials, we'll explore critical information that will enable you to handle a variety of emergency care situations.

The chapter has been designed to help you make timely emergency medical decisions. Under each condition, we'll address the appropriate care to provide and we'll also note what type of professional medical assistance, if any, is necessary.

We encourage you to keep this information handy. You can trust that the material in this chapter, and the book as a whole, has been painstakingly written and reviewed by physicians and health experts. You're armed with credible, reliable information that has the power to save lives.

ONE ESSENTIAL QUESTION…

When Do I Need to Call 911?

CALL 911 IF:

✓ The victim's condition is life-threatening

✓ The victim is unconscious

✓ The victim is unable to breathe

✓ Moving the victim may cause further harm

✓ Transportation to the emergency room is unavailable or would take too long

✓ The victim is bleeding severely

✓ The victim is in shock

✓ The victim has been poisoned

✓ The victim asks you to call

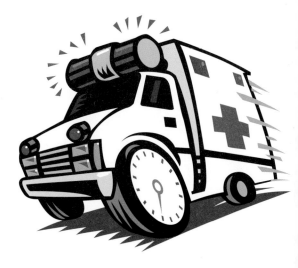

HOW TO TREAT...

Bites & Stings

There are several types of bites that can inflict harm. Animal, human, insect, snake, and spider bites will be addressed in this chapter. The important thing to remember when providing aid to a bitten person is that bites can be serious and deserve immediate attention. While most bites can be treated without the assistance of medical personnel, there are many circumstances where professional help should be sought out.

CALL 911 IF:

- You believe you have been bitten by a poisonous animal
- The wound is bleeding severely and the flow of blood cannot be stopped

SEE A DOCTOR IF:

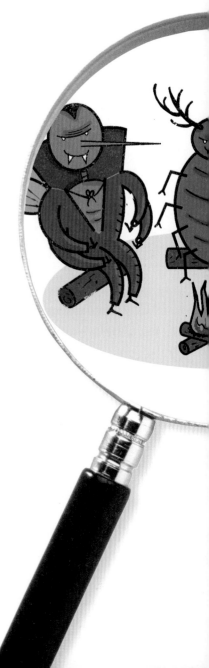

- The bite came from a wild animal (rabies is highly possible)
- The bite came from a domesticated animal that was acting strangely, was foaming at the mouth, or attacked without reason
- You are bitten by a domesticated animal whose owner cannot be located or cannot verify that the animal has been vaccinated for rabies
- The bite came from a cat or human (infection is highly possible)
- The bite is severe and may need stitches
- The bite is to the face, hands, or feet
- The wound becomes infected—signs of infection include the following:
    - ✓ Heat or red streaks extending away from the wound
    - ✓ Liquid discharge coming from the wound
    - ✓ Fever, swelling, redness, or tenderness

"Dogs that bark at a distance never bite."

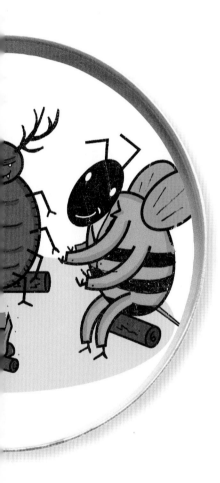

TREATING WITH SELF-CARE

■ **Care for the wound**

✓ Clean the bite or sting immediately with warm water and soap (if stung, the stinger may need to be removed first)

✓ Refer to the "Scrapes, Cuts, and Punctures" section (p.22) and treat the wound as directed

✓ Apply ice to the bite or sting if swelling occurs

✓ For tick bites, remove the tick with tweezers by grasping as close to the skin as possible and pulling straight back

■ **Prevent further damage**

✓ Verify that the bite did not come from a poisonous or rabid animal

✓ If you suspect the bite came from a poisonous or rabid animal, call 911 immediately

✓ Verify that the victim's rabies vaccinations are current

✓ If you note swelling, redness, or itching, take an oral antihistamine or apply calamine lotion to relieve the itching

PREVENTING BITES & STINGS

■ Vaccinate all pets against rabies

■ Do not keep wild animals as pets

■ Teach kids not to play with stray pets

■ Avoid and teach your kids to avoid any contact with wild animals

■ Never disturb any animal (domesticated or wild) while it is eating or caring for its young

HOW TO TREAT...

Burns

When it comes to burns, prevention is critical. Typically, prevention takes the form of fire/smoke detectors, fire extinguishers, as well as cooking and other safety precautions.

But before we look at the detailed aspects of prevention, we need to consider what to do if prevention efforts fail and a burn occurs. The first step is to determine what degree of burn has occurred. This is done by observing the depth of the burn.

There are 3 basic types of burns:

1 **First-Degree Burns.** A first-degree burn affects only the outer layer of skin (epidermis) and is generally treatable as a minor burn with self-care remedies. The skin will be dry, red, and painful to the touch. A sunburn is a good example of a first-degree burn.

2 **Second-Degree Burns.** A second-degree burn involves multiple layers of skin. The burned area typically becomes blistered, swollen, and may weep or leak fluid.

3 **Third-Degree Burns.** Third-degree burns involve all layers of the skin and will likely damage underlying tissue and/or organs. These burns are often less painful because nerves have been destroyed. The skin may be charred black, or will have a dry, white or yellowish appearance.

Once the degree of burn has been determined, it is time to determine what, if any, medical attention is needed.

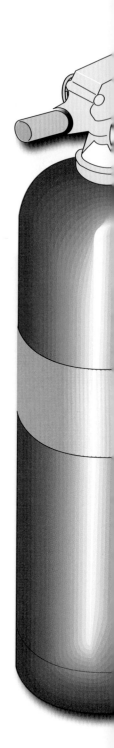

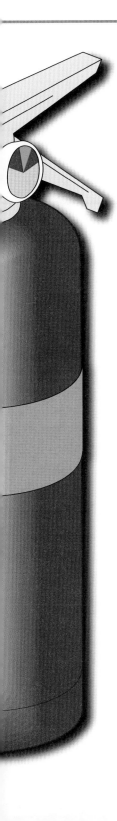

CALL 911 IF:

- It is a third-degree burn (DO NOT attempt to treat a third-degree burn or remove clothing that is stuck to the burned area)
- The burn is a second-degree or third-degree burn that involves the head, hands, feet, or genitals
- The burn is a second-degree burn that is larger than 1 inch in diameter
- The burn involves a child, elderly person, pregnant person, or individual with a weakened immune system
- A strong chemical (e.g., acid, lye, etc.) is splashed in an eye

SEE A DOCTOR IF:

- A burn becomes infected—signs of infection may include the following:
  - ✓ Heat or red streaks extending away from the wound
  - ✓ Liquid discharge coming from the wound
  - ✓ Fever, swelling, redness, or tenderness
- A strong chemical burn occurs on a large portion of the body or on the face
- An eye appears damaged after home treatment from a chemical burn
- Pain does not subside in a chemically burned eye after 20 minutes of home treatment
- A child, elderly person, pregnant person, or individual with a weakened immune system gets sunburned over a large portion of their body

Continued on next page...

HOW TO TREAT...

Burns

TREATING WITH SELF-CARE

■ **Provide initial care**

✓ Extinguish the source of the burn, if possible

✓ Make sure there is no smoldering material still on the victim

✓ To reduce pain and swelling, use large amounts of cool water or apply a cool, sterile bandage/cloth for at least 10 minutes (DO NOT use ice or ice water on a burn)

✓ Have the victim lie down to help prevent shock

✓ Make sure the victim is breathing

✓ With first-degree and second-degree burns, remove rings, belts, and other constrictive clothing to allow for swelling

■ **Provide follow-up care**

✓ Do not apply cold treatments for too long a period

✓ Keep the area uncovered and elevated when possible

✓ Apply a dry dressing, if necessary

✓ Avoid using anesthetic sprays and creams, oils, greasy ointments, and/or butter—these can slow the healing process and may cause an allergic reaction

✓ Use aloe vera on first-degree and second-degree burns to ease pain and promote healing

✓ Do not break blisters

✓ Take aspirin or ibuprofen to help relieve pain

✓ Call your doctor if you show signs of infection after 2 days (odor, pus, and/or extreme redness)

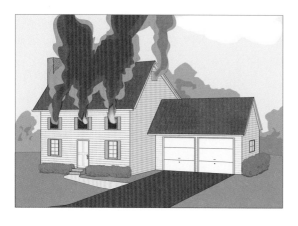

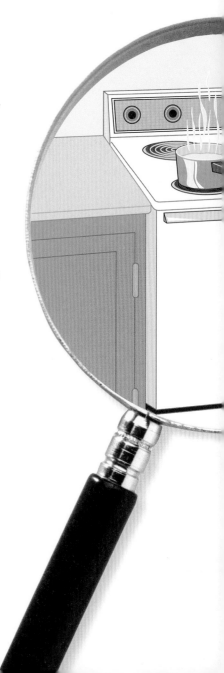

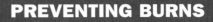
PREVENTING BURNS

■ **At home**

✓ Install smoke detectors on all floors of your home or apartment (check the batteries in smoke detectors twice a year)

✓ Keep a fire extinguisher in your home, preferably near the kitchen

✓ Have an established plan for exiting your house or apartment should a fire occur—make sure that everyone in your family is familiar with the plan

✓ Set your water heater no higher than 120°F

■ **While working**

✓ Wear appropriate clothing and eye protection when working with flammable materials

✓ Practice safety when working in the kitchen (e.g., turn pot handles in toward the middle of the stove, supervise children closely, etc.)

✓ Read labels on all household cleaning products and lawn chemicals carefully

■ **During play**

✓ Practice sun safety (e.g., always wear sunscreen, avoid the sun during the peak hours of 10 a.m. to 2 p.m., etc.)

✓ Wear UV protective sunglasses and clothing

✓ When staying with friends, relatives, or in a hotel, make sure to acknowledge the fire escape plan before going to sleep for the night

✓ Use extreme caution with campfires and cookouts

WORDS TO THE WISE

Most fatal fires occur at night while families are asleep. Check the batteries in your smoke detectors twice a year. Smoke detectors save lives!

HOW TO TREAT...

Choking

Choking occurs when the airway is blocked in the throat or windpipe. The condition is potentially life-threatening and should be given attention immediately.

CALL 911 IF:

- You are unable to clear the victim's airway
- The victim loses consciousness
- The choking victim is an infant or elderly person

SEE A DOCTOR IF:

- The victim is stable, but lost consciousness for a time
- The victim sustained injury during the choking spell

TREATING WITH SELF-CARE

HELPING CONSCIOUS VICTIMS

- **Know when NOT to help**
  - ✓ DO NOT begin choking rescue procedures if the victim CAN speak, cough, or breathe—instead, encourage the victim to continue coughing

- **Clear the airway**
  - ✓ If the victim CANNOT speak, cough, or breathe, give abdominal thrusts (the Heimlich maneuver) as follows:
    - Get behind the victim and reach around their abdomen
    - Position 1 clenched fist just under the rib cage in the middle of the abdomen, with the thumb against the abdomen
    - Grasp your clenched fist with your other hand and pull back and upward under the rib cage quickly and sharply
    - Continue thrusts until the object is dislodged

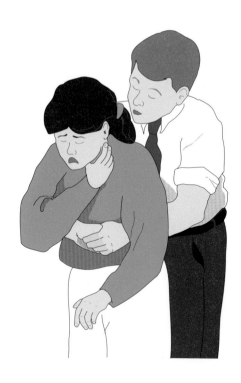

TREATING WITH SELF-CARE

HELPING UNCONSCIOUS VICTIMS

■ **Clear the airway**

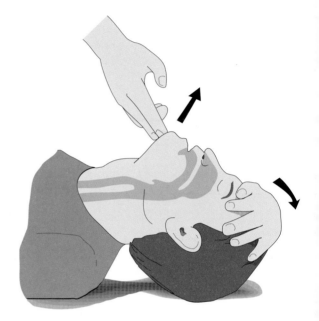

✓ Lower the victim to the ground and place them flat on their back

✓ Tilt the victim's head and open their mouth

✓ Look, listen, and feel for breathing

✓ If the victim is still not breathing, refer to the "Unconscious" section (p. 28) and provide breathing care—before giving a breath, look for an object in the throat and if seen, remove it

✓ If you are unable to clear the airway, continue with this sequence referred to in the "Unconscious" section

✓ If the airway has been cleared, continue with rescue breathing and/or chest compressions as necessary (See p.28-30)

Continued on next page...

"DO NOT begin choking rescue procedures if the victim CAN speak, cough, or breathe—instead, encourage the victim to continue coughing."

HOW TO TREAT...

Choking

HELPING CONSCIOUS INFANTS

■ **Call for help!**

   ✓ If an infant is choking, call 911 immediately

■ **Perform back blows**

   ✓ Place the infant face down on your forearm (their head should be supported by your hand and slightly lower than the rest of their body)

   ✓ Rest your forearm on your thigh

   ✓ Deliver 4 distinct, forceful blows with the heel of your hand between the infant's shoulder blades

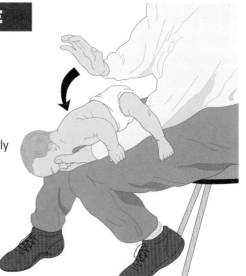

■ **Perform chest thrusts**

   ✓ After 4 back blows, grasp the infant between your forearms and rotate the infant onto their back

   ✓ Using your top hand, position 2 fingers on the lower part of the infant's breastbone in the middle of the abdomen, and give 4 distinct upward thrusts, depressing the breastbone 1/2 to 1 inch

   ✓ Inspect the infant's mouth for foreign objects and perform a finger sweep of the mouth only if an object is visible

HELPING UNCONSCIOUS INFANTS

■ **Continue to attempt to clear the airway**

   ✓ Repeat the sequence of back blows, chest thrusts, and mouth inspections until the object is dislodged or help arrives

■ **Provide rescue breathing**

   ✓ After each sequence, check for signs of breathing

   ✓ If necessary, attempt rescue breathing as detailed in the "Unconsciousness" section (p.28-30)

   ✓ Watch for the infant's chest to rise if the airway has been cleared

   ✓ If the airway has been cleared, continue with rescue breathing and/or chest compressions as necessary (See p.28-30)

WORDS TO THE WISE

Depend on others for help. Let them know you need help by bringing your hands up to your neck. And, under no circumstances should you leave others and go to the restroom! You could find yourself in a life-threatening situation without anyone to help.

TREATING WITH SELF-CARE

HELPING YOURSELF

■ **Perform chest thrusts**

    ✓ If you are alone and begin choking, position 1 clenched fist just under the rib cage in the middle of the abdomen, with the thumb against the abdomen

    ✓ Grasping your clenched fist with your other hand, pull back and upward under the rib cage quickly and sharply

    ✓ Perform 4 distinct thrusts, attempting to dislodge the object

■ **Call for help**

    ✓ If you are unable to dislodge the object after 4 thrusts, call 911 immediately (if unable to speak, just dial and set down the phone—they will trace the call)

■ **Perform aided chest thrusts**

    ✓ After calling 911, press your upper abdomen over the back of a chair or any firm object and use the weight of your body to perform 1 firm thrust

    ✓ Repeat this procedure until the object is dislodged

PREVENTING CHOKING

■ Chew food slowly and fully

■ Don't speak with food in your mouth

■ Use extra caution if you have false teeth

■ Keep objects that will fit into a young child's mouth out of reach

■ Avoid driving with food, a toothpick, or other foreign objects in your mouth

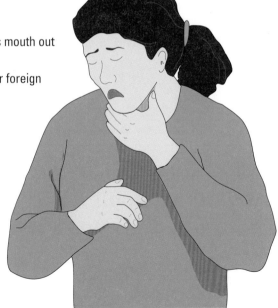

HOW TO TREAT…

Drowning

Drowning occurs when a person suffocates as a result of being submerged in water or another liquid. If the airway is not cleared and breathing restored, the victim will die.

In examining this emergency from a self-care point of view, it's important to first consider when it is appropriate to seek professional medical assistance.

CALL 911 IF:

- You see a drowning victim (e.g., a person waving their hands, shouting for help, struggling to stay above water, etc.)
- You have rescued a victim, but there is no breathing or no pulse
- You suspect a head or neck injury

SEE A DOCTOR IF:

- A person has blue lips and ears or cold, pale skin after a near-drowning incident
- A person develops a fever or cough after a near-drowning incident
- A person develops muscle pain after a near-drowning incident

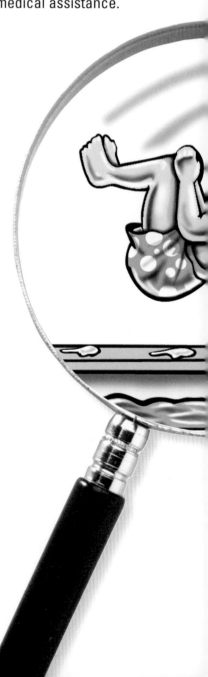

"Make sure all neighborhood swimming pools have adequate fences and gates."

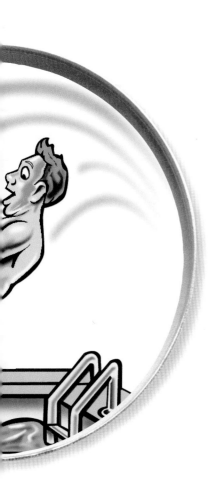

TREATING WITH SELF-CARE

- Get the drowning victim out of the water
- If the victim is unconscious, look, listen, and feel for breathing and a pulse (See p.28)
- If the victim is not breathing or has no pulse, refer to the "Unconsciousness" section of this book for aid (p.27)
- Remove cold, wet clothes and warm the victim with dry blankets, clothing, or personal body heat
- If you suspect head or neck injuries, don't move the victim once out of the water (immobilize the head by wrapping rolled towels or articles of clothing on either side of the neck)

PREVENTING DROWNING

- **Take precautions**
  - ✓ Make sure all neighborhood swimming pools have adequate fences and gates
  - ✓ Tell your child to never swim alone
  - ✓ Never walk or ice-skate on untested ice
  - ✓ Never leave a young person alone near any amount of water or in the bathroom
- **Be prepared**
  - ✓ Make sure you and your family have taken swimming lessons
  - ✓ If you are responsible for supervising kids at the pool, learn CPR
  - ✓ Teach your children to always check the depth of the water before diving in
  - ✓ Practice safe boating by bringing along enough life jackets and avoiding alcohol

HOW TO TREAT...

Head Injury

The vast majority of head injuries are treatable at home and do not require emergency medical care. However, more serious head injuries can be life-threatening. Here's what to look for.

CALL 911 IF:

- You suspect spine or neck injury
- The victim is bleeding severely or bleeding/leaking clear, watery fluid from the ears or nose
- The victim has bruising or discoloration behind the ears or around the eyes
- The victim has no pulse or is not breathing
- The victim's skull has an abnormal deformity, is swollen, or has depressions
- The victim remains unconscious for more than 3 minutes
- The victim is unable to move their arms or legs

SEE A DOCTOR IF:

- The victim loses consciousness for less than 3 minutes
- The victim experiences loss of memory, dizziness, or vomiting
- The victim experiences a prolonged headache, nausea, and/or enlarged or unequal pupils

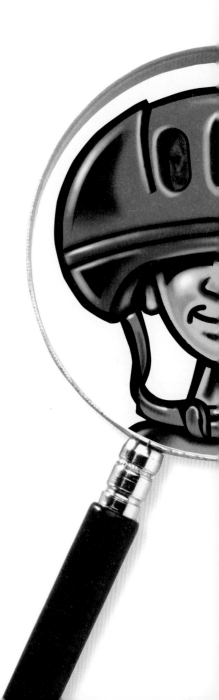

"Always wear protective head gear when participating in sporting events such as football, boxing, baseball, and horseback riding."

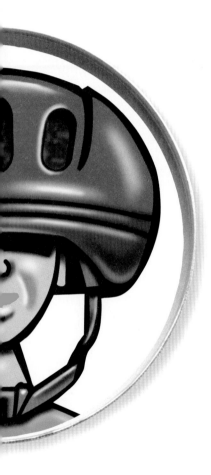

TREATING WITH SELF-CARE

■ **Observe the victim**

✓ Keep the victim lying down in a dimmed room

✓ Apply ice to the injured area to reduce swelling or bruising (do not put ice directly on the skin)

✓ Carefully monitor the victim's vital signs

✓ If the victim loses consciousness, provide the appropriate care as detailed in the "Unconsciousness" section of this book (p.27)

■ **Treat other conditions**

✓ Care for any scrapes, cuts, or punctures that may have occurred as a result of the injury (See p.22)

✓ Observe the victim for signs of shock and provide care as detailed in the "Shock" section of this book (p.26)

PREVENTING HEAD INJURY

■ Always wear protective headgear when participating in sporting events such as football, boxing, baseball, and horseback riding

■ Always wear protective headgear when riding two-wheel vehicles such as bicycles and motorcycles

■ Always wear protective headgear when working in construction zones that require this precaution

■ Always wear your seatbelt and have passengers wear their seatbelts

■ Keep stairs free of clutter

■ Use extra caution when walking on wet or slippery surfaces

HOW TO TREAT...

Heat Exhaustion & Heatstroke

Heat exhaustion can be a common occurrence given the right region of the country and the right time of year. Typically this condition, although potentially serious, does not require professional medical assistance. The primary symptoms of heat exhaustion are listed below.

SYMPTOMS OF HEAT EXHAUSTION

■ Fatigue, headache, nausea, and general weakness
■ Cold, moist, or pale skin

The greatest danger of heat exhaustion is that it can quickly become heatstroke. Heatstroke is far more serious and requires immediate medical attention. Below is some information to help you know when to call for help.

CALL 911 IF:

■ You suspect the victim's heat exhaustion has become heatstroke—signs of heatstroke include the following:

✓ Rapid or weak heartbeat

✓ Rapid or shallow breathing

✓ No sweating and/or hot, red, dry skin

✓ Dilated pupils

✓ Convulsions, nausea, and/or loss of consciousness

✓ Very high temperature (104°F or higher)

SEE A DOCTOR IF:

■ The victim maintains a medium grade fever
■ The victim has non-stop vomiting
■ The victim has pale, cool, and/or clammy skin
■ The victim is too dizzy or weak to stand

TREATING WITH SELF-CARE

■ **Cool down and re-hydrate**

✓ Move the victim out of the sun and into a cool place

✓ Loosen the victim's clothing

✓ Give the victim a sponge bath with cool water

✓ Make sure the victim drinks some fluids immediately and continually over the course of the next 24 hours (8 to 16, 8-ounce glasses of water should be consumed per day)

✓ Give the victim salty foods to help them retain water

■ **Watch for heatstroke**

✓ Monitor the victim for signs of heatstroke

✓ If the victim does not start to feel better after 15 to 20 minutes, get professional help

PREVENTING HEAT EXHAUSTION & HEAT STROKE

■ **Play it safe**

✓ Avoid direct sun exposure during peak hours (10 a.m. to 2 p.m.)

✓ Avoid strenuous physical activity during hot or humid weather

✓ Avoid heavy meals when spending time outside in hot weather

✓ Wear light-colored clothing that is lightweight and breezy

✓ Bring and drink at least 1 liter of water for every 1 1/2 hours you're out in the sun

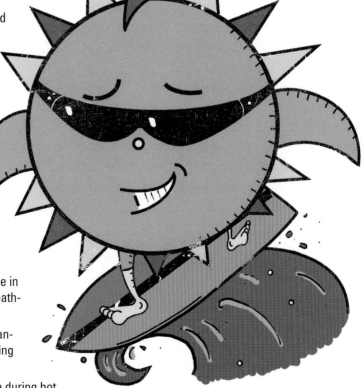

■ **Use your head**

✓ Never stay or leave anyone in parked cars during hot weather—this includes pets

✓ Never bundle babies in blankets or heavy clothing during hot weather

✓ Avoid alcohol and caffeine during hot weather

HOW TO TREAT...

Poisonings

Each year, millions of people are accidentally poisoned. Victims most commonly come in contact with a poisonous product in the kitchen, the bathroom, or the garage, but a poisoning can take place anywhere.

A call to the Poison Control Center should typically be the first step in care.

CALL POISON CONTROL IF:

- You have good reason to suspect a poisoning—signs of a poisoning include the following:
    - ✓ Open or spilled bottles of medication or other toxic substances
    - ✓ Chemical burns on the victim's lips, nose, mouth, or clothing
    - ✓ Vomiting, sleepiness, fever, chills, difficulty breathing, dizziness, weakness, confusion, seizures, or muscle twitches

CALL 911 IF:

- The victim is unconscious
- The victim has stopped breathing
- The victim has no pulse

SEE A DOCTOR IF:

- Your Poison Control Representative advises you to do so

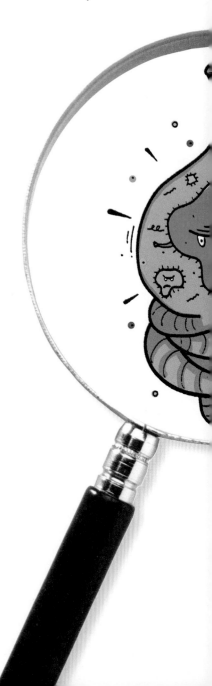

"If you or someone you know has been poisoned, call your local Poison Control Center immediately."

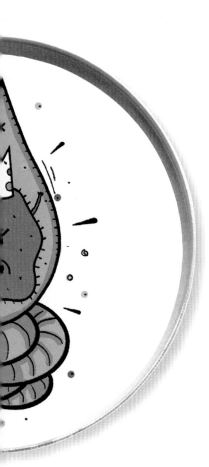

TREATING WITH SELF-CARE

- **Call your Poison Control Center and tell them:**
  - ✓ What substance was taken
  - ✓ How much of the substance was taken
  - ✓ How long ago the substance was taken
  - ✓ Whether or not the victim has vomited
  - ✓ The age, gender, weight, condition, and any medical problem(s) of the victim
- **Follow the advice of the Poison Control Representative**

PREVENTING POISONINGS

- **Play it safe**
  - ✓ Lock up poisonous substances
  - ✓ Store all medications and poisonous substances in their original marked containers
  - ✓ Make sure all medications are stored in childproof containers
  - ✓ Properly destroy and dispose of all unused and/or expired medications (call your pharmacist for details)
  - ✓ Keep children away from lead-based chemicals such as paint chips and lead water pipes
  - ✓ Purchase syrup of ipecac to induce vomiting and activated charcoal for absorption when recommended
- **Get outfitted**
  - ✓ Wear protective gear when handling chemicals and dangerous substances
  - ✓ Install a carbon monoxide detector in your home
  - ✓ Know your local Poison Control Center's telephone number

Continued on next page...

KEYING IN ON...

Food Poisoning

One of the more common forms of poisoning is food poisoning. Symptoms include nausea, vomiting, diarrhea, and stomach pain.

TREATING WITH SELF-CARE

■ **Seek professional medical help when:**
- ✓ The victim is less than 6 months old and is vomiting
- ✓ The victim has chest pain or a fever
- ✓ The bowel movements or vomit of the victim are black or bloody
- ✓ The victim's symptoms last longer than 48 hours
- ✓ You suspect that medications are the underlying cause of the symptoms

■ **Provide the proper care**
- ✓ Have the victim consume several glasses of water every hour for as long as the vomiting and/or diarrhea lasts
- ✓ Once vomiting/diarrhea has stopped, begin feeding the victim clear liquids, such as broth, and mild foods including applesauce, mashed bananas, and white rice

PREVENTING FOOD POISONING

■ Keep foods hot or cold—room temperature is where many bacteria grow

■ Set your refrigerator between 34°F and 40°F

■ Defrost meats in the refrigerator or microwave

■ Never leave meats sitting on the counter

■ Keep your kitchen clean—clean countertops are especially important

■ Cook hamburger and other ground meats thoroughly

■ Don't eat uncooked or raw eggs

■ Throw away canned or jarred foods with leaks

■ Don't eat foods that have been left out for 2 hours or longer

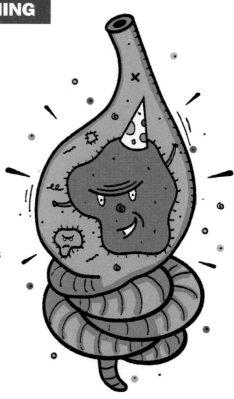

HOW TO TREAT...

Roadside Emergencies

In this day and age, we spend a lot of time in the automobile and travel great distances every year. Unfortunately, accidents and injuries on the road are a reality. Here are some things to keep in mind if you should be involved in one of these unfortunate circumstances.

TREATING WITH SELF-CARE

■ **Assess the scene**
- ✓ Start by assessing the scene for safety
- ✓ Secure the scene so that no further injuries are likely to take place

■ **Assess the victims**
- ✓ Assess all victims so that aid can be given first where it is needed most
- ✓ Make sure that someone has called 911 and provided comprehensive information as to the conditions of the victims and the scene

■ **Employ the help of others**
- ✓ Trained individuals should provide aid to injured persons
- ✓ Individuals without training should facilitate traffic and monitor safety
- ✓ Additional individuals should provide comfort to victims

■ **Provide appropriate care**
- ✓ Refer to appropriate sections within this book for the care of victims
  - ■ "Unconsciousness" (p.27)
  - ■ "Scrapes, Cuts, & Punctures" (p.22)
  - ■ "Shock" (p.26)

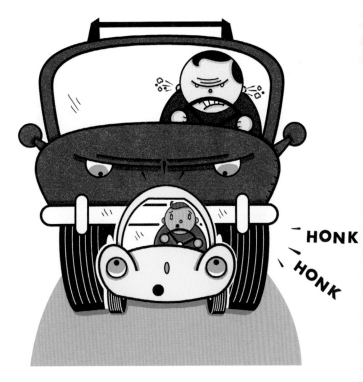

HONK
HONK

HOW TO TREAT...

Scrapes, Cuts, & Punctures

Scrapes, cuts, and punctures are potentially serious injuries that warrant immediate attention. The first step in treating one of these injuries is identifying the type of injury.

Scrapes. A scrape damages the surface of the skin and is also referred to as an abrasion.

Cuts. A cut slices the skin and is also referred to as a laceration.

Punctures. A puncture wound is caused by the penetration or stabbing of an object into the skin.

CALL 911 IF:

- The wound is to the head, neck, chest, or abdomen and is serious
- You are unable to slow the bleeding by applying pressure for 15 minutes
- An object is stuck in a wound in a vital area (i.e., head, neck, chest, or abdomen)
- The person goes into shock—refer to the "Shock" section for signs and treatment (p.26)
- The victim's skin near the wound is discolored and cold, or there is tingling, numbness, loss of feeling, or an inability to move the limb beyond the wound

SEE A DOCTOR IF:

- The wound requires stitches (i.e., it is bleeding severely)
- A wound gets infected—signs of infection may include the following:
  - ✓ Heat or red streaks extending away from the wound
  - ✓ A liquid discharge from the wound
  - ✓ Swelling, redness, tenderness, or a fever

TREATING WITH SELF-CARE

INITIAL CARE FOR SCRAPES & CUTS

■ **Clean the wound**

✓ Thoroughly wash the wound with warm water and soap

■ **Stop the bleeding**

✓ Attempt to stop the bleeding by applying direct pressure with a bandage for 15 minutes

✓ Repeat 15-minute pressure periods as needed

✓ If the initial 15-minute period of direct pressure does not result in any noticeable slowing of bleeding, see a doctor while maintaining pressure and elevation

✓ If bleeding has not stopped completely after 3, 15-minute pressure cycles (45 total minutes of pressure) see a doctor

FOLLOW-UP CARE FOR SCRAPES & CUTS

■ **Allow the scrape or cut to heal**

✓ Apply antibiotic ointment and cover the wound with a sterile bandage

✓ Apply a new, clean bandage at least once a day or when the bandage gets wet or damaged

■ **Prevent further damage**

✓ If the wound becomes infected, schedule an appointment with your doctor

✓ If you are not sure when your last tetanus vaccination was, call your doctor as soon as possible (tetanus boosters should be received within 48 hours of the injury, if needed)

Continued on next page...

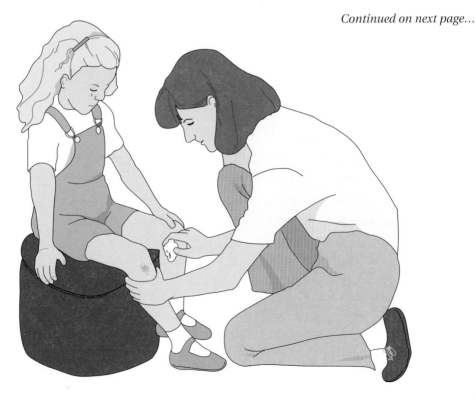

HOW TO TREAT…

Scrapes, Cuts, & Punctures

TREATING WITH SELF-CARE

INITIAL CARE FOR PUNCTURES

■ **Clean the wound**

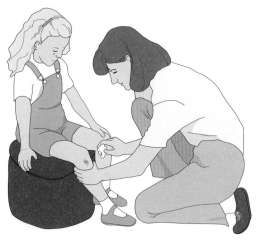

- ✓ Remove the object if the puncture is not a serious one to the head, neck, chest, or abdomen (call 911 in these instances)
- ✓ Clean the wound thoroughly with warm water and soap

■ **Stop the bleeding**

- ✓ If there is continued bleeding, elevate the site of the wound
- ✓ Attempt to stop the bleeding by applying direct pressure with a bandage for 15 minutes
- ✓ Repeat 15-minute pressure periods as needed
- ✓ If the initial 15-minute period of direct pressure does not result in any noticeable slowing of bleeding, see a doctor while maintaining pressure and elevation
- ✓ If bleeding has not stopped completely after 3, 15-minute pressure cycles (45 total minutes of pressure) see a doctor

FOLLOW-UP CARE FOR PUNCTURES

■ **Allow the puncture to heal**

- ✓ Apply antibiotic ointment and cover the wound with a sterile bandage
- ✓ Apply a new, clean bandage at least once a day or when the bandage gets wet or damaged

■ **Prevent further damage**

- ✓ If the wound becomes infected (e.g., odor, pus, and/or extreme redness), schedule an appointment with your doctor
- ✓ If you are not sure when your last tetanus vaccination was, call your doctor as soon as possible (tetanus boosters should be received within 48 hours of the injury, if needed)

HOW TO TREAT...

Seizures

Normal brain functions are impaired during a seizure, causing the cells of the brain to behave in abnormal ways. Only in the rarest of seizure cases is a call to 911 warranted. However, seeing a doctor may often be in order.

CALL 911 IF:

- The victim has stopped breathing, has no pulse, or is unconscious
- The victim suffers a serious injury during the seizure
- The seizure is a first-time occurrence
- The seizure occurred in an infant younger than 6 months old
- The seizure lasts longer than 5 minutes
- The victim is pregnant

SEE A DOCTOR IF:

- The victim received a wound during the seizure that requires attention
- The victim's doctor has requested to be informed of all seizures

TREATING WITH SELF-CARE

- **During the seizure**
  - ✓ Do not hold or restrain the person
  - ✓ Clear as many objects from the person's path as possible to prevent injury
  - ✓ Loosen tight clothing around the head and neck
  - ✓ Roll the victim on their side to help drain any fluids from the mouth
  - ✓ Do not place anything in the victim's mouth
- **After the seizure**
  - ✓ Comfort the victim once the seizure has ended
  - ✓ Check for injuries once the seizure has ended
  - ✓ Ask bystanders not to crowd the victim

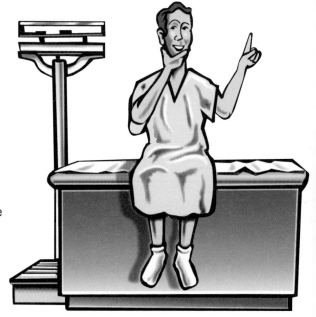

HOW TO TREAT...

Shock

Shock can result from various conditions. Some of these conditions include traumatic injuries, severe heat, infections, poisonings, blood loss, and/or poor circulation.

SIGNS AND SYMPTOMS

- A shock victim may be conscious or unconscious
- Pale, gray, cool, and/or clammy skin
- Weak or rapid pulse
- Slow or shallow breathing
- Low blood pressure
- Weakness or trembling
- Over-excitement or anxiety
- Nausea or vomiting
- Enlarged pupils

CALL 911 IF:

- Someone is in shock—emergency medical personnel should always be called immediately in cases of shock

TREATING WITH SELF-CARE

- Have the person lie down on their back
- Elevate the feet above the level of the head with pillows, blankets, or other available objects
- Loosen tight clothing and cover the victim with a blanket
- Keep the victim from moving unnecessarily
- Do not give the victim anything to drink
- If the victim is vomiting, turn them on their side to avoid choking
- Comfort the victim until emergency medical personnel arrive

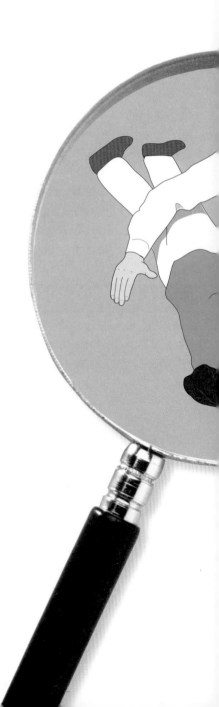

HOW TO TREAT...

Unconsciousness

Emergency situations that involve a loss of consciousness are always life-threatening. Many lives could be saved if more of us were armed with the right information.

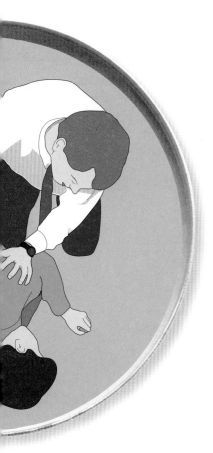

CALL 911 IF:

- The victim is unconscious, not breathing, or has no pulse
- You suspect that the victim has injured their neck or spine
- The victim is bleeding severely
- The victim goes into shock
- A victim regains breathing capacity and/or a pulse after losing it for a time

SEE A DOCTOR IF:

- A victim's condition stabilizes

ASSESS THE SCENE

- If the emergency scene is on a highway, interstate, or roadway, consider traffic first and foremost
- If the emergency scene involves dangerous equipment (e.g., power lines, machinery, etc.), make sure the danger posed by the equipment is controlled before offering help
- If the emergency scene involves a lake, pool, or other body of water, make sure when offering help that you are equipped with adequate floatation devices

Continued on next page...

"Many lives could be saved if more of us were armed with the right information."

HOW TO TREAT...

Unconsciousness

TREATING WITH SELF-CARE

PROVIDE AIRWAY CARE

■ Determine if the victim is unconscious—
if so, shout for help and have someone
call 911 immediately

■ Carefully position the victim flat on their
back (if you suspect spine or neck injury, do
not move the victim unless there is a serious danger at the present scene)

■ Tilt the chin up and the head back, opening
the victim's airway

■ Look, listen, and feel for breathing

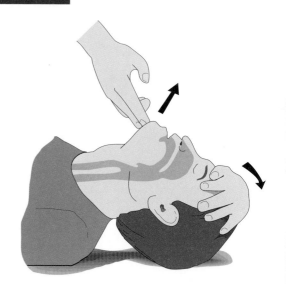

PROVIDE BREATHING CARE

■ With the victim's head tilted, place 1 of your
hands on the victim's forehead, also using
your thumb and forefinger to pinch closed
the victim's nose

■ Use your other hand to support the victim's
head by placing it under their chin

■ After inhaling a deep breath, place your
mouth over the victim's mouth, creating a
tight seal, and slowly and fully exhale,
taking 1 1/2 to 2 full seconds to exhale
completely

■ During the breath, watch and note whether
the victim's chest rises

  ✓ If the chest does rise, proceed with a
  second full breath

  ✓ If the chest does not rise, the victim's
  airway may be obstructed—refer to the
  "Choking" section for details (p.8)

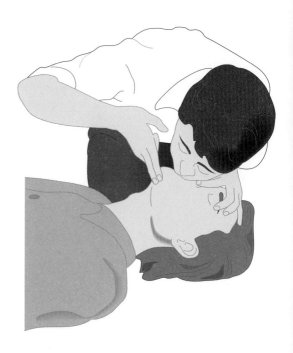

TREATING WITH SELF-CARE

PROVIDE CIRCULATION CARE

■ **The position**

- ✓ Use your fingers to locate the bottom (closer to the waist) of the victim's breastbone and place 2 fingers at this point
- ✓ Using your free hand, place the heel of your palm above your 2 placed fingers (closer to the victim's head)
- ✓ Place the hand used to identify the bottom of the breastbone on top of your other placed hand
- ✓ Interlock and raise your fingers off the victim's chest
- ✓ Lock your elbows and position your shoulders directly above your placed hands

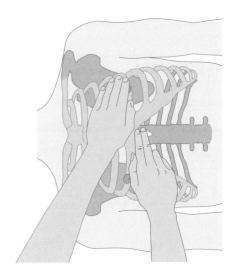

PROVIDE BREATHING CARE

■ **The procedure**

- ✓ Use the weight of your body to rhythmically compress the victim's chest 1 1/2 to 2 inches
- ✓ Complete 15 compressions, never unlocking your elbows or raising your hands off the victim's chest
- ✓ Count aloud to maintain appropriate rhythm ("1 and 2 and 3 and 4 and…")
- ✓ Once 15 compressions have been completed, repeat the 2-breath procedure indicated in the breathing instructions
- ✓ After completing 4 cycles of compressions and breaths, repeat the procedure described above for checking breathing and pulse
- ✓ If breathing is not present, repeat the aid just described

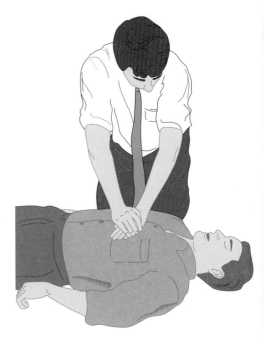

Continued on next page…

HOW TO TREAT...

Unconsciousness

CARE FOR INFANTS AND SMALL CHILDREN

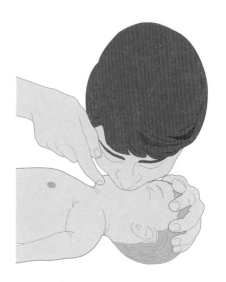

PROVIDE AIRWAY CARE

■ **Small Children**

✓ Follow the same care presented for adults

■ **Infants**

✓ Don't tilt the head back more than one or two inches

✓ Proceed as you would with an adult

PROVIDE BREATHING CARE

■ **Small Children**

✓ Follow the same care presented for adults

✓ Exhale for only 1 to 1 1/2 seconds

■ **Infants**

✓ Cover both the mouth and nose, forming a tight seal

✓ Exhale for only 1 to 1 1/2 seconds

PROVIDE CIRCULATION CARE

■ **Small Children**

✓ Use only the heel of 1 hand to compress the chest

✓ Compress the chest between 1 and 1 1/2 inches at a rate of 80 to 100 compressions per minute

✓ Give 1 breath for every 5 compressions

■ **Infants**

✓ Use only two fingers of one hand to compress the chest

✓ Use your free hand to support the back of the infant during compressions

✓ Compress the chest 1/2 to 1 inch at least 100 times per minute

✓ Give 1 breath for every 5 compressions

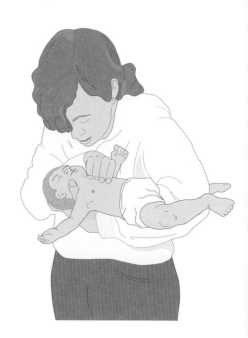

CHAPTER TWO:

Our Most Common Conditions

There's no question that a few common conditions consume the bulk of the medical expense dollar. These are the conditions that, for whatever reason, plague us and drive us in droves to seek medical care.

In this chapter of Self-Care Essentials, we'll look at these conditions and offer some legitimate solutions. Where appropriate, these solutions will serve as alternatives to unnecessary professional medical care and expense.

ALTERNATIVES... NOT REPLACEMENTS

It's important that we make one point crystal clear: we're not suggesting that professional medical care is totally unnecessary—in fact, it's often needed. What we are saying is that too often we seek medical assistance when we could treat the problem on our own. We just need to be empowered with reliable information.

That's the aim of this chapter—to provide credible health information in an easy-to-understand format that eliminates all the mystery from our most common conditions. These are real solutions that will safeguard your health and the health of your family.

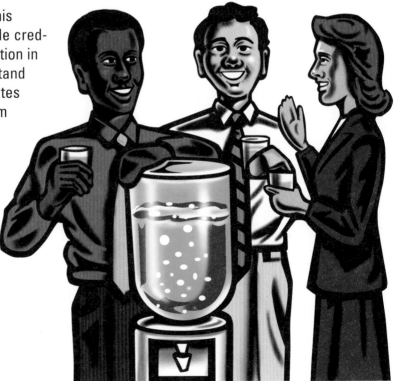

HOW TO TREAT...

Asthma, Bronchitis, & Hay Fever

Asthma is a condition in which there is a narrowing of the airways often brought on by an allergic reaction. Bronchitis is a chronic or temporary inflammation and constriction of the air passages in the lungs. Hay fever is a severe, acute allergic reaction in the upper respiratory system and eyes. The first step in care for these three conditions is to identify the nature of the problem.

SIGNS AND SYMPTOMS

■ **Asthma & Bronchitis**
- ✓ A deep cough
- ✓ Yellowish-gray, green, or bloody mucus discharged from the lungs
- ✓ Wheezing in cold weather
- ✓ Difficulty breathing
- ✓ Strain or pull on the neck, chest, or ribs while breathing
- ✓ Difficulty talking or performing other tasks
- ✓ Bluish skin discoloration, especially on the lips
- ✓ Light-headedness
- ✓ Symptoms that worsen at night

■ **Hay Fever**
- ✓ Coughing
- ✓ Sneezing
- ✓ Excessive production of mucus
- ✓ Stuffy or runny nose
- ✓ Itchy eyes, nose, or throat
- ✓ Fatigue

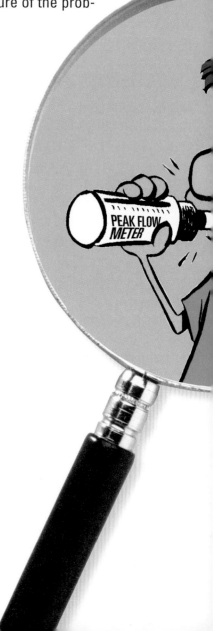

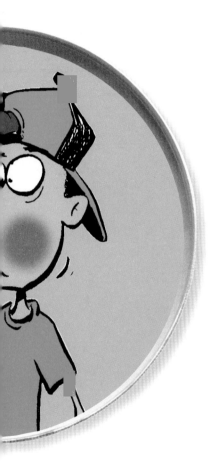

TREATING WITH SELF-CARE

■ **Asthma**

✓ There is no cure for asthma, but it is very treatable

✓ Make sure you have a peak flow meter, learn how to use it, and use it regularly

✓ Drink 8 to 16, 8-ounce glasses of water per day

✓ Establish an asthma reaction plan with your doctor—broad aspects of the plan should include:

 ▪ Stay calm when an attack occurs

 ▪ Stop whatever activity you may be doing at the first sign of an attack

 ▪ Sit up straight and breathe slowly and easily

 ▪ Use your inhaler to open your airway (inhalers can mask severe attacks—be careful and know your condition)

 ▪ Keep a diary of your condition, noting all relevant prevention, attack, and treatment information

■ **Bronchitis**

✓ Get plenty of rest

✓ Drink 8 to 16, 8-ounce glasses of water per day

✓ Use a humidifier in your home and keep this device clean

✓ Use aspirin, ibuprofen, or acetaminophen to help relieve body aches and fever

✓ Don't smoke and avoid secondhand smoke

■ **Hay Fever**

✓ Take antihistamines to treat allergic reactions

✓ Take decongestants to reduce congestion and/or inflammation in the nasal passageway

✓ Use nasal sprays to treat allergic reactions

Continued on next page...

HOW TO TREAT...

Asthma, Bronchitis, & Hay Fever

SEE A DOCTOR IF:

■ **Asthma**
- ✓ You are having a great deal of difficulty breathing
- ✓ You experience strain or pull on the neck, chest, or ribs while breathing
- ✓ Your medications have not relieved your symptoms after 20 minutes
- ✓ You are having symptoms that indicate heart trouble, such as chest pain
- ✓ You are coughing up yellow, green, or bloody matter
- ✓ It is your first attack
- ✓ You start relying on your medication more and more
- ✓ You have an attack and medication is not available
- ✓ You notice a bluish skin discoloration, especially on the lips

■ **Bronchitis**
- ✓ The bronchitis lasts for more than 3 days
- ✓ You continue to cough up matter from your lungs for more than 10 days
- ✓ The matter becomes yellow, green, or bloody
- ✓ You experience severe, labored breathing or significant pain while breathing
- ✓ You become dehydrated or are unable to eat foods
- ✓ You experience a fever for longer than 2 days
- ✓ An infant, older adult, or chronically ill person shows signs or symptoms of bronchitis

■ **Hay Fever**
- ✓ You cannot breathe well enough to talk
- ✓ You experience severe wheezing
- ✓ Mucus discharge is yellow, green, or bloody
- ✓ You feel like you're going to pass out
- ✓ Your symptoms interfere with daily activities
- ✓ Your lips, tongue, or face are swollen or blue
- ✓ You develop a rash, itching, or increased body temperature

PREVENTING ASTHMA, BRONCHITIS, & HAY FEVER

■ **Be smart**

 ✓ Know your allergies

 ✓ Avoid allergens that trigger symptoms

 ✓ Use available devices such as the furnace, air conditioner, dehumidifier, and/or humidifier to control allergens, pollens, and molds and be sure to keep these devices clean

 ✓ Avoid air irritants such as smoke and strong odors

 ✓ Control cockroaches (cockroaches are known to trigger symptoms)

 ✓ Avoid strenuous activities in cold, dry environments

 ✓ Wear a scarf over your mouth and nose when out in cold weather

■ **Do the right thing**

 ✓ Strictly follow the advice of your doctor

 ✓ Take medications only as prescribed

 ✓ Wear a mask when working outside or around allergens

 ✓ Reduce stress and fatigue

 ✓ Get at least 30 minutes of exercise most days of the week

 ✓ Consider building immunity through allergy shots

 ✓ Keep your bedding clean

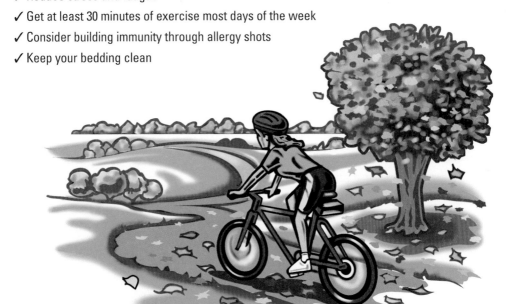

HOW TO TREAT...

Chest Pain

Heart attacks, angina, pulmonary embolisms, indigestion/heartburn, and chest muscle pain are all different kinds of chest pain. These conditions range from minor to life-threatening. The first step is identifying the seriousness of the problem.

SIGNS & SYMPTOMS OF SERIOUS CONDITIONS

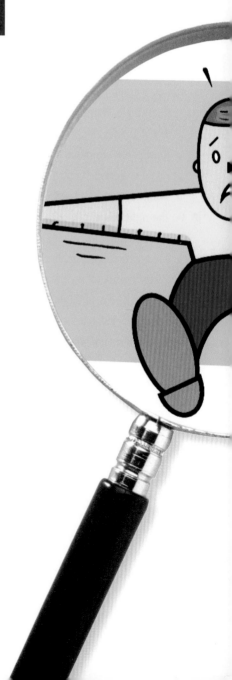

- **Heart attacks** (interruption of blood supply to the heart)
  - ✓ A burning, crushing, and/or squeezing pain or pressure in the chest
  - ✓ Pain in the arms, neck, back, and/or jaw
  - ✓ Pain that doesn't go away or lasts longer than 15 minutes
  - ✓ Irregular pulse or heartbeat
  - ✓ Nausea, vomiting, shortness of breath, dizziness, weakness, sweating
- **Angina** (a lack of enough oxygen to the heart)
  - ✓ Pressure or pain in the heart that comes and goes
  - ✓ Feeling of numbness or heaviness behind the breastbone
  - ✓ Pain that spreads to the upper back, neck, jaw, or shoulders
  - ✓ Pain that is relieved by resting or taking prescribed medication
- **Pulmonary Embolism** (a blood clot in the lung)
  - ✓ Chest pain with sudden shortness of breath
  - ✓ Pain in breathing, especially deep breathing
  - ✓ Anxiety, fear, or a sense of impending doom
  - ✓ A rapid heartbeat
  - ✓ Coughing up bloody matter

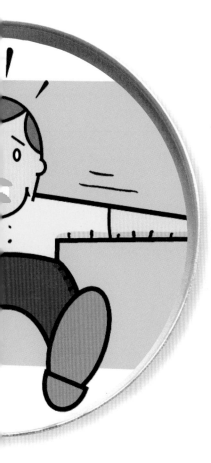

SIGNS & SYMPTOMS OF MINOR CONDITIONS

- Heart palpitations (i.e., uneven or fast heartbeat)
- Pain that follows a heavy or spicy meal
- Pain that is sensitive or painful to the touch (i.e., chest muscle strain)

TREATING WITH SELF-CARE

SERIOUS CONDITIONS

- **Heart Attacks & Pulmonary Embolisms**
  - ✓ Call 911
  - ✓ Do not go to a place to be alone and rest
  - ✓ Do not ignore the warning signs—early treatment is the best recourse

- **Angina**
  - ✓ Lie down and rest
  - ✓ Make sure someone is with you in person or on the phone
  - ✓ Have a developed plan of action for attacks
  - ✓ Take medications as prescribed

MINOR CONDITIONS

- **Indigestion or Heartburn**
  - ✓ Take over-the-counter medications such as antacids
  - ✓ Try to breathe slowly and deeply in an upright position
  - ✓ Avoid caffeine, mints, chocolate, and citrus fruits

- **Chest Muscle Pain**
  - ✓ Apply ice, a topical ointment, or a pain reliever to reduce pain
  - ✓ Avoid activities that may further stress or strain the area

Continued on next page...

HOW TO TREAT...

Chest Pain

SEE A DOCTOR IF:

■ Your symptoms indicate a heart attack or pulmonary embolism—call 911

■ Your symptoms of angina do not subside after 15 minutes—call 911

■ Your symptoms are new or more severe

■ Your indigestion is severe, frequent, or seems uncontrollable

■ Your stools are very dark

■ Chest muscle pain does not improve after 1 week

PREVENTING CHEST PAIN

■ Get at least 30 minutes of exercise most days of the week

■ Eat a well-balanced, low-fat diet

■ Avoid spicy foods and late night eating

■ Don't smoke and avoid secondhand smoke

■ Reduce stress

■ Have your blood pressure and cholesterol checked regularly

■ Know your family's history of heart disease

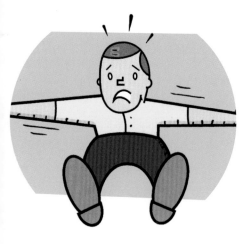

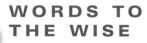

WORDS TO THE WISE

Any chest pain you experience that is new or different is worth a visit to your doctor. Schedule an appointment as soon as possible.

HOW TO TREAT...

Depression

First things first, depression is treatable! The condition is described in general terms as a feeling of sunken spirits. It plagues millions and can range from a minor problem to a life-threatening illness.

Depression can be caused by any of a number of concerns in a person's life. Some common causes include: drug and alcohol abuse, high levels of stress, other serious medical conditions, medication side effects, and possibly an inherited genetic trait.

SIGNS AND SYMPTOMS

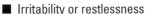

- Feelings of sadness or hopelessness
- Fatigue
- Lack of concentration
- Crying spells
- Loss of interest in previously enjoyed activities
- Changes in eating and sleeping patterns
- Thoughts of suicide or death
- Frequent aches and pains that don't respond to treatment
- Irritability or restlessness

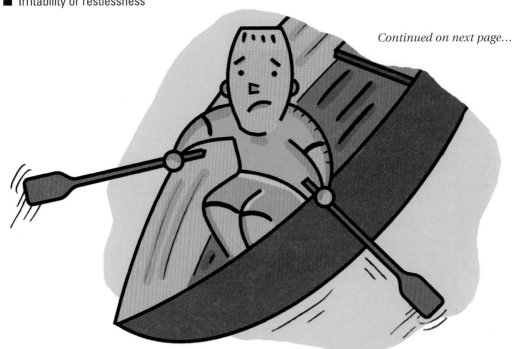

Continued on next page...

HOW TO TREAT...

Depression

TREATING WITH SELF-CARE

■ See a doctor if your depression lasts longer than 6 weeks or is severe—strictly follow their advice

■ Don't overwork yourself

■ Avoid making major life decisions when feeling depressed

■ Avoid using alcohol or non-prescribed drugs

■ Spend time with people

■ Get adequate sleep

■ Get at least 30 minutes of exercise most days of the week

SEE A DOCTOR IF:

■ You feel suicidal or act violently

■ You hear voices encouraging harmful behavior

■ You suffer significantly or repeatedly from any of the symptoms for no known reason

■ Periods of grieving last for more than 4 weeks

■ Your behavior changes suddenly

■ You believe your symptoms are related to a medication you're taking

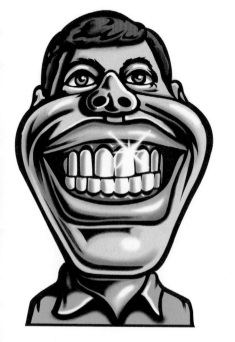

WORDS TO THE WISE

It is extremely important to remember that depression can be treated, no matter what the cause. If you or someone you know suffers from depression, try multiple solutions—sooner or later one solution is bound to get the sufferer smiling again.

HOW TO TREAT...

Digestive Disorders

Diarrhea, nausea and vomiting, and constipation are common disorders that can affect the digestive system. Digestive disorders can occur at any point along the digestive tract. They typically result in pain and discomfort. The first step is identifying the problem.

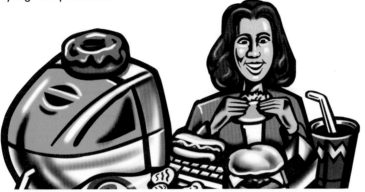

SIGNS AND SYMPTOMS

■ **Diarrhea**
- ✓ More than 3 or 4 loose, watery stools per day
- ✓ Often accompanied by abdominal cramps

■ **Nausea & Vomiting**
- ✓ Queasy and/or dizzy sensation
- ✓ Weak and sweaty feeling

■ **Constipation**
- ✓ Difficult passage of hard stools 3 or fewer times per week
- ✓ A bloated sensation
- ✓ Cramping and abdominal discomfort

TREATING WITH SELF-CARE

■ **Diarrhea**
- ✓ Avoid high-fiber and solid foods until symptoms subside
- ✓ Drink 8 to 16, 8-ounce glasses of water per day
- ✓ Avoid specific foods such as dairy, fats, and spicy foods for several days
- ✓ Avoid caffeine, don't smoke, and avoid secondhand smoke
- ✓ Try over-the-counter antidiarrheals after 12 hours

Continued on next page...

HOW TO TREAT...

Digestive Disorders

TREATING WITH SELF-CARE

■ **Constipation**

- ✓ Use a mild laxative, but do not rely on laxatives for long periods
- ✓ Increase the amount of daily fiber consumption
- ✓ Consider taking a fiber supplement
- ✓ Drink 8 to 16, 8-ounce glasses of water per day
- ✓ Get at least 30 minutes of exercise most days of the week

■ **Nausea & Vomiting**

- ✓ Stop eating and drinking for several hours
- ✓ Try ice chips and/or sips of liquid to avoid dehydration
- ✓ Return to solid and/or high-fiber foods slowly as nausea and vomiting clear
- ✓ Avoid specific foods such as dairy, fats, and spicy foods for several days
- ✓ Try soda crackers, clear soups, gelatin, or rice to avoid hunger

SEE A DOCTOR IF:

■ **Diarrhea**

- ✓ Diarrhea lasts longer than 1 week
- ✓ You become dehydrated—symptoms of dehydration include little or no urination, weakness or dizziness, an excessively dry mouth
- ✓ Your stools are bloody
- ✓ A fever of 101.5°F or higher occurs with the diarrhea

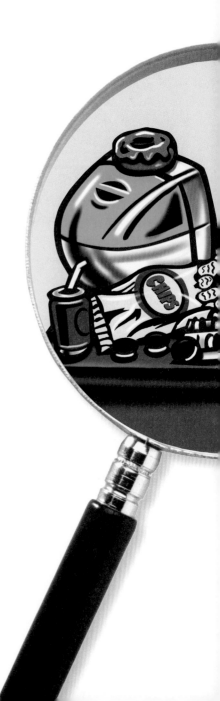

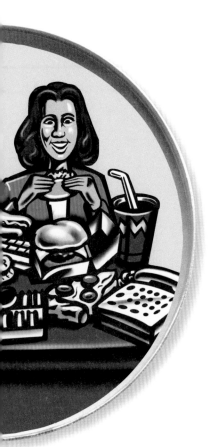

SEE A DOCTOR IF:

■ **Constipation**

   ✓ Constipation lasts longer than 3 weeks

   ✓ You experience bleeding with stools

   ✓ You rely on laxatives to have bowel movements

■ **Nausea & Vomiting**

   ✓ Symptoms last longer than 3 days

   ✓ Vomiting with a fever lasts longer than 2 days

   ✓ Your vomit contains blood

   ✓ You become dehydrated

   ✓ Vomiting is triggered from medications

PREVENTING DIGESTIVE DISORDERS

■ Don't eat foods you suspect may be spoiled

■ Thoroughly wash all utensils and food service/preparation products

■ Wash hands regularly and always before eating

■ Don't smoke and avoid secondhand smoke

■ Avoid too much caffeine and/or alcohol

■ Drink 8 to 16, 8-ounce glasses of water per day

■ Eat plenty of fiber

■ Get at least 30 minutes of exercise most days of the week

■ Always pass bowel movements as soon as possible

"To eat is human to digest is divine."

– MARK TWAIN

HOW TO TREAT...

Fatigue

For millions of Americans, fatigue is more than a daily annoyance—it's a life-altering condition that lowers productivity and drains ambition. Eliminating fatigue is something most sufferers can do at home with the right information. The first step is identifying the problem.

SIGNS AND SYMPTOMS

- Loss of energy and/or appetite
- Mood changes
- Problems sleeping
- Depression and/or an inability to focus
- Sleepiness
- Weakness
- Difficulty remembering
- General aches and pains

TREATING WITH SELF-CARE

- **Change your environment**
  - ✓ Get out of the house and go for a drive or walk
  - ✓ Open a window and let in some fresh air
  - ✓ Turn on some music
- **Change your activities and your mood**
  - ✓ Spend time with your family
  - ✓ Get plenty of sleep
  - ✓ Avoid excessive television viewing
  - ✓ Engage in meaningful dialogue with your family and friends
  - ✓ Treat and eliminate negative emotions
  - ✓ Monitor and eliminate conditions such as high blood pressure

SEE A DOCTOR IF:

- You suspect your fatigue is related to medication
- You suspect your fatigue is related to depression or other psychological conditions
- Your fatigue is severe and limits your usual activities for longer than 2 weeks
- Symptoms worsen despite efforts to eliminate fatigue
- You begin to lose weight and have not changed your diet or exercise
- Your fatigue is accompanied by a sore throat, swollen glands, abdominal pain, or other suspected illnesses

PREVENTING FATIGUE

- **Say yes to:**
  - ✓ At least 30 minutes of exercise most days of the week
  - ✓ Eating a well-balanced diet
  - ✓ Monitoring the effects of medications
  - ✓ Good relationships with people
  - ✓ Standing up to stretch often
  - ✓ Proper lighting and air ventilation
  - ✓ Doing something in the evenings, like a hobby
  - ✓ Making house tasks fun and involving everyone
- **Say no to:**
  - ✓ Excessive alcohol and caffeine
  - ✓ Tobacco
  - ✓ Excess weight
  - ✓ Doing the same thing all day
  - ✓ Plopping down on the couch the instant you get home from work

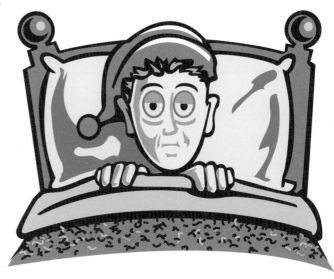

HOW TO TREAT...

Fever

A normal body temperature ranges between 97°F and 100°F. A body temperature above 100°F indicates a fever. Detecting a fever is fairly straightforward. For best results, you may want to consider using a digital thermometer with disposable plastic probe covers.

Here's the rest of what you need to know.

SIGNS AND SYMPTOMS

- General feeling of illness
- Flushed appearance
- Skin that feels warm to the touch
- Chills or cold sweats

TREATING WITH SELF-CARE

- Drink 8 to 16, 8-ounce glasses of water per day
- Eat foods easy to digest, such as soup
- Get plenty of rest
- Take acetaminophen, aspirin, or ibuprofen to reduce your fever
- Take a sponge bath with lukewarm (not cold) water (do not use rubbing alcohol)

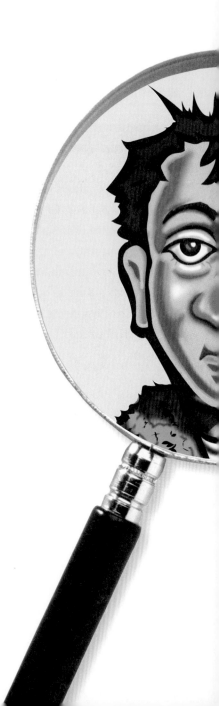

*"A temperature of 101.5°F or higher is a **treatable fever**. This means you should call a doctor and follow their advice."*

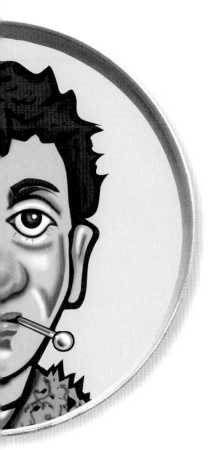

SEE A DOCTOR IF:

- A fever is 101.5°F or higher (this is a treatable fever, call a doctor and follow their advice)
- A fever is accompanied by any of the following:
  - ✓ Seizures, confusion, or extreme irritability
  - ✓ Abnormal breathing
  - ✓ Pain or stiffness in the neck
  - ✓ Sore throat, vomiting, diarrhea, painful urination, and/or earaches
- The person is less than 6 months old
- A fever lasts longer than 4 days in adults or longer than 2 days in children
- The person has recently undergone surgery of any kind
- A fever occurs after having traveled out of the country
- A fever occurs after taking a new medication

PREVENTING FEVERS

- Drink 8 to 16, 8-ounce glasses of water per day
- Get at least 30 minutes of exercise most days of the week
- Wash hands regularly and thoroughly
- Eat a well-balanced diet
- Try to get 8 hours of sleep per night
- Reduce stress

HOW TO TREAT...

Frostbite

Frostbite occurs when the skin and underlying tissues freeze. Any part of the body can get frostbitten, but the hands, feet, nose, and ears are the most susceptible. The first step is identification.

SIGNS AND SYMPTOMS

- A tingling or numb sensation
- Pain in the affected area
- Swelling
- White skin
- Loss of function in the affected area
- Skin that feels hard and solid
- Blisters on the affected area

TREATING WITH SELF-CARE

- Get inside or take shelter from the wind
- Loosen and remove wet and/or tight clothing
- Don't rub the affected area(s)
- Slowly thaw the affected area(s) for 45 minutes to 1 hour as follows:
  - ✓ Soak in a tub of warm water, just above body temperature
  - ✓ Use blankets or coats to thaw
  - ✓ Press the affected area(s) against other warm parts of the body
- Elevate the affected area(s)
- Use additional caution to protect the area(s) from the cold until it is completely healed
- If blisters form, do not purposefully break them

"Wear multiple layers of clothing in cold weather with the outer layer being wind and water repellant."

SEE A DOCTOR IF:

- Skin swells and becomes solid
- The victim loses function in the affected area(s)
- The skin turns red or purple
- The victim experiences memory loss
- Numbness remains after thawing the area(s)

PREVENTING FROSTBITE

- Wear multiple layers of clothing in cold weather with the outer layer being wind and water repellant
- 1 thick sock is best for keeping your feet warm
- Always wear gloves or mittens and a hat that covers the ears
- Avoid alcohol and tobacco
- Shield your face and hands from the wind

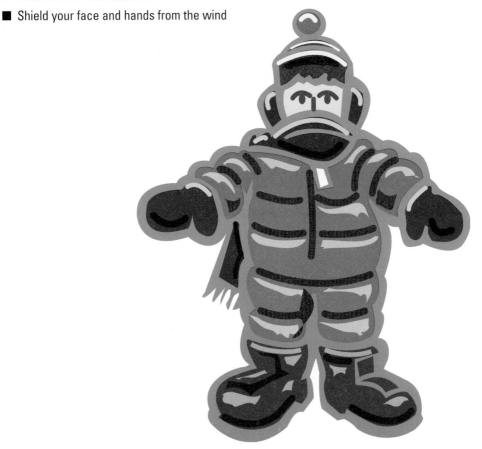

HOW TO TREAT...

General Aches & Pains

Backaches, earaches, headaches, sprains and strains, and toothaches are all addressed in this broad category. These are the injuries and annoyances that occur so frequently and that we typically just muddle through. But, there is self-care we can employ to lessen the pain and speed healing. The first step in care is to identify the problem.

SIGNS AND SYMPTOMS

- Pain or a dull ache in specific areas of the body
- Stiffness and/or lack of mobility in a specific area of the body
- Acute tension in areas of the body
- Knotted or tight muscles
- Fatigue

TREATING WITH SELF-CARE

- Apply ice to bruises and swollen areas of the body
- Elevate injured or painful parts of the body above the level of the heart
- Take an over-the-counter medication to relieve the pain
- Get adequate rest, but stay cautiously active—prolonged rest causes muscles to weaken
- Carefully and gently massage affected muscles
- For strains and sprains, wrap the area with a snug elastic bandage (remove the bandage every several hours for a few moments to restore normal blood flow)
- Gargle warm water with salt for a toothache

"Self-care can lessen the pain and speed the healing of general aches and pains."

SEE A DOCTOR IF:

■ Backaches

✓ The pain is severe

✓ The pain came on suddenly and without an identifiable cause

✓ You have difficulty moving the injured area

✓ You experience numbness or tingling in one of your extremities

✓ You are an older adult (over 60)

✓ Pain does not start to go away after 1 week of self-care

✓ You have involuntary movements/spasms

✓ You become unable to control urination or bowel movements

✓ You also experience abdominal pain at the same time

✓ You notice a cracking sound in the affected area during movement

■ Earaches and Headaches

✓ The pain began due to a blow to the head

✓ You also experience a stiff neck, fever, drowsiness, nausea, or vomiting

✓ You begin to experience difficulty hearing

✓ Your ear seeps sticky or bloody discharges

✓ You also experience a clicking when opening and shutting the mouth

✓ Your pupils appear large

✓ Your vision is blurred or doubled

✓ Your speech is slurred

✓ The pain lasts for longer than 3 days

✓ You suspect the pain is related to medication

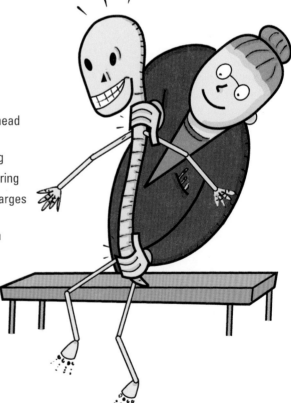

Continued on next page...

HOW TO TREAT...

General Aches & Pains

IDENTIFYING...
Headaches

Check out the various types of common headaches below.

Tension headaches are often associated with anxiety, nervous tension, and the contraction of scalp muscles. The pain is usually a steady, not throbbing, ache affecting both sides of the head.

Migraines are severe, recurring headaches often accompanied by vision disorders and nausea. The pain is usually a throbbing pain felt on one side of the head.

Sinus headaches are caused by a blockage of the sinus cavity and are, contrary to popular belief, quite rare.

SEE A DOCTOR IF:

■ **Sprains and Strains**
- ✓ The pain seems to get worse with time
- ✓ Swelling and/or pain is severe
- ✓ You become unable to move the injured area
- ✓ The injured area loses color and/or feeling
- ✓ The bones around the injured area seem to protrude in an unusual or new manner
- ✓ There is a clicking feeling or sound when the injured area is moved
- ✓ The injury occurred with great force

■ **Toothaches**
- ✓ The pain spreads to the lower jaw, neck, chest, or arms
- ✓ You begin to sweat with the occurrence of the pain
- ✓ You also have a fever
- ✓ Your gums are red, swollen, or bleeding
- ✓ Your face swells
- ✓ Your toothache keeps you awake or wakes you up

PREVENTING ACHES & PAINS

■ **Exercise correctly**
- ✓ Always stretch thoroughly before exercise
- ✓ Use protective athletic apparel
- ✓ Don't over-do it

■ **Be good to your teeth**
- ✓ Brush and floss twice a day
- ✓ Visit the dentist every 6 months
- ✓ Limit sweets in your diet
- ✓ Chew sugar-free gum after meals when you can't brush

PREVENTING ACHES & PAINS

■ **Practice good lifting techniques**

✓ Stand close to the object

✓ Place your feet securely and squarely about a shoulder's width apart

✓ Keep your back as straight as you can with your knees bent

✓ Lift slowly with your legs bearing as much of the weight as possible

✓ Keep your head tilted up (like you're looking at the ceiling) when lifting

✓ Use a back brace for heavy or repeated lifting

■ **Live smart**

✓ Get at least 30 minutes of exercise most days of the week

✓ Eat a well-balanced diet

✓ Try to get 8 hours of sleep per night

✓ Reduce stress

✓ Get in the habit of stretching every day

✓ Sleep on a firm mattress with your back supported

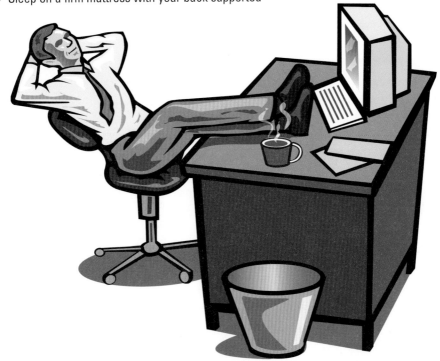

HOW TO TREAT...

Premenstrual Syndrome

Premenstrual syndrome is a group of symptoms brought on by normal changes in women's hormone levels. The symptoms take place during the 2-week period after ovulation (release of an egg) and before menstruation.

SIGNS AND SYMPTOMS

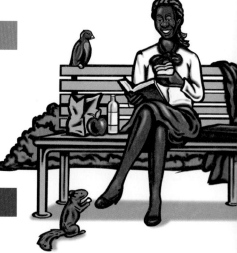

- Weight gain
- Soreness in the breasts and/or dull body aches
- Bloating/fluid retention, especially in the hands and feet
- Fatigue, depression, irritability, and/or hostility
- Nausea and vomiting, diarrhea, and/or constipation
- Food cravings

TREATING WITH SELF-CARE

- Try eating smaller meals
- Limit alcohol and caffeine and eliminate tobacco
- Use relaxation techniques to control emotional discomforts
- Take over-the-counter medication to treat symptoms

SEE A DOCTOR IF:

- Your emotional symptoms are severe or long-lasting
- Your symptoms prohibit you from accomplishing necessary tasks
- Any of your symptoms last longer than the 2-week premenstrual time period
- You feel powerless to improve the symptoms you suffer from

PREVENTING PMS

- Maintain an appropriate weight—not too low or too high
- Eat a well-balanced diet
- Take a multi-vitamin/mineral
- Get at least 30 minutes of exercise most days of the week
- Limit the amount of salt in your diet
- Know your symptoms and predict their arrival

HOW TO TREAT...

Respiratory Conditions

Colds, sinusitis, coughs, sore throats, and the flu are all conditions that occur in the respiratory system. These conditions share many of the same causes—viral or bacterial infections, allergies, air pollutants, and nasal congestion.

SIGNS AND SYMPTOMS

■ **Colds and Flu**

- ✓ Runny nose, sneezing, and nasal congestion
- ✓ Sore throat
- ✓ Headache
- ✓ Cough
- ✓ Fever
- ✓ Fatigue
- ✓ Aches and pains

■ **Sinusitis**

- ✓ Fever
- ✓ Nasal obstruction and difficult breathing
- ✓ Pain in the upper jaw, eyes, cheeks, and/or facial tissues of the nose
- ✓ Headache
- ✓ Nasal and/or head congestion and drainage
- ✓ Yellowish-green nasal drainage

■ **Sore Throats and Coughs**

- ✓ Scratchy, dry feeling in the throat
- ✓ Sneezing
- ✓ Pain when swallowing
- ✓ A mild fever
- ✓ Raspy voice
- ✓ Nasal drainage and postnasal drip

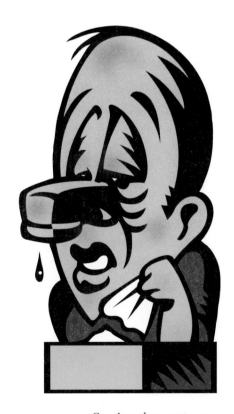

Continued on next page...

HOW TO TREAT...

Respiratory Conditions

TREATING WITH SELF-CARE

- Drink lots of warm drinks to soothe the throat, loosen congestion, and flush your system
- Get plenty of rest
- Take over-the-counter medications to reduce pain and lower fevers
- Take lozenges or cough drops to soothe sore throats
- Gently blow your nose regularly
- Avoid milk and other dairy products, which may cause mucus to thicken
- Use the prevention tips listed in this section to avoid spreading the condition
- Use a humidifier or a cool mist vaporizer and clean these devices often

PREVENTING RESPIRATORY CONDITIONS

- Wash your hands often and always before eating—use warm water and soap for a minimum of 30 seconds
- Keep your hands away from your face
- Avoid close contact with persons with respiratory conditions
- Get plenty of rest
- Get at least 30 minutes of exercise most days of the week
- Eat a well-balanced diet
- Use a tissue when you sneeze and encourage others to do the same
- Use a humidifier through winter months and clean the device often
- Consider an annual flu shot

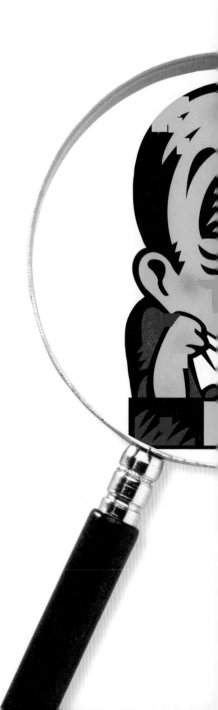

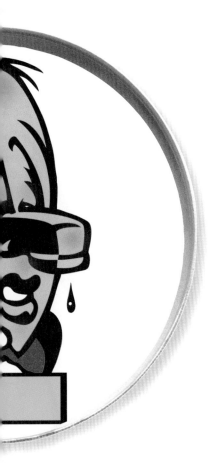

■ **You have:**

✓ A fever

✓ Swollen glands in your neck

✓ A skin rash

✓ Vomiting, abdominal pain, or chest pain

✓ Confusion or delirium

✓ Pain or swelling in your sinuses that changes when you move your head

✓ Chest, neck, jaw, or arm pain

✓ Side effects from any of the medications you may be taking

■ **You notice that:**

✓ Your urine is dark in color

✓ You are having difficulty getting enough oxygen

✓ Your tonsils are bright red or have white spots on them

✓ You are coughing up mucus that is yellow, green, or gray

✓ Your breath, throat, nose, or ears smell bad even after washing

✓ You are coughing up blood

■ **Your symptoms:**

✓ Do not start to improve after 1 week

✓ Do not cease completely after 2 weeks

✓ Continue to get worse with time

HOW TO TREAT...

Skin Disorders

Skin disorders don't have to be a mystery. Acne, athlete's foot, and eczema are three common skin disorders that can easily be improved with proper care. Here's the information you need to know in order to combat and prevent these conditions.

SIGNS AND SYMPTOMS

- **Acne**
  - ✓ Raised bumps (pimples) of bacteria and secretions under the skin on the face, chest, shoulders, or upper back
  - ✓ Bumps may appear white, black, or red
- **Athlete's Foot**
  - ✓ Itchy feet and/or redness between the toes
  - ✓ Cracked skin on the feet between the toes
  - ✓ Wet scales, especially between the toes
  - ✓ Blisters on the feet and between the toes
- **Eczema (Atopic Dermatitis)**
  - ✓ Itchy, red, raised rash on the face, scalp, neck, bend of the elbows or knees, buttocks, thighs, or torso
  - ✓ Blister-like, crusty scales

"Skin disorders don't have to be a mystery. They can easily be improved with proper care."

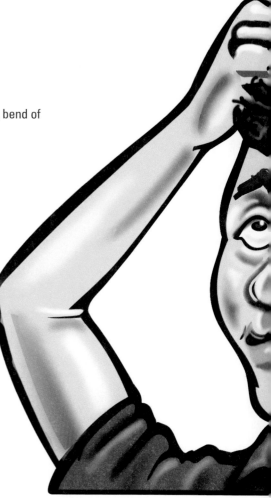

TREATING WITH SELF-CARE

■ **Acne**

- ✓ Leave your skin alone—popping the pimples will lead to infections and scarring
- ✓ Wash your face with warm water, soap, and a clean washcloth
- ✓ Try over-the-counter medications

■ **Athlete's Foot**

- ✓ Use over-the-counter antifungal powders, lotions, and sprays
- ✓ Follow the prevention tips presented in this section

■ **Eczema**

- ✓ Avoid over-drying your skin with long, hot baths and/or showers
- ✓ Use only mild soap on the affected areas
- ✓ Use lotion after showers to keep your skin lubricated
- ✓ Leave the affected area alone—don't scratch it

Continued on next page…

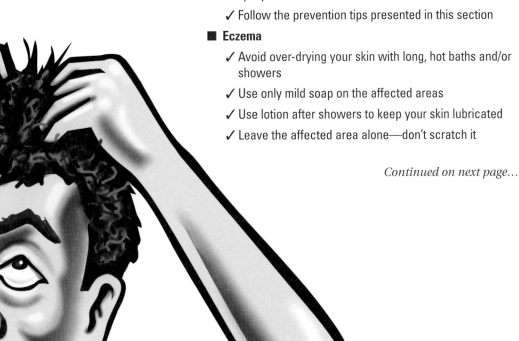

HOW TO TREAT...
Skin Disorders

SEE A DOCTOR IF:

■ You have signs of infection, such as redness surrounding the area, swelling, or a fever

■ Your acne is severe and you are unable to improve it with home treatment

■ The pimples are large and painful

■ You are suffering from athlete's foot and you have problems with circulation

■ You are also diabetic

■ You have a large amount of weeping or crusting with your eczema

■ The rash lasts for longer than 2 weeks

■ The eczema interferes with your sleep

PREVENTING SKIN DISORDERS

■ **Acne**

✓ Wash thoroughly using a washcloth with a mild soap

✓ Try over-the-counter medications such as degreasing pads that have benzoyl peroxide in them

✓ Keep your hair clean and off your face

✓ Avoid excessive sun exposure and artificial tanning bulbs

✓ Don't use oily or cream-based lotions or makeup

✓ Eat a well-balanced diet

✓ Reduce stress

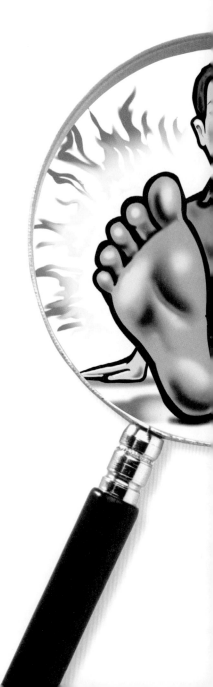

PREVENTING SKIN DISORDERS

■ **Athlete's Foot**

- ✓ Keep your feet dry and clean
- ✓ Carefully wash and dry between the toes twice a day
- ✓ Wear sandals or thongs in public showers
- ✓ Wear cotton socks to absorb moisture

■ **Eczema**

- ✓ Avoid wool fabrics
- ✓ Wash with a mild soap after sweating
- ✓ Reduce stress
- ✓ Limit your consumption of foods such as eggs, milk, seafood, or wheat products
- ✓ Be careful to note any products or substances that you may be allergic to
- ✓ Use a humidifier in your home and clean the device often

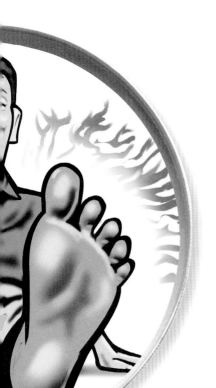

WORDS TO THE WISE

Skin disorders often require a coordinated effort between a sufferer and a physician. This is especially true for the prescription of needed medications. If your self-care treatment is ineffective, consider consulting a professional.

HOW TO TREAT...

Urinary Tract Infections

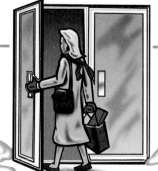

Urinary tract infections are caused by a bacterial infection. The bacterial infection can be in the kidneys, the passageway between the kidneys and the bladder (ureter), the bladder itself, or in the passageway out of the body (urethra).

SIGNS AND SYMPTOMS

- A strong or frequent need to urinate
- Burning, pain, or bleeding during urination
- Chills, fever, nausea, or vomiting
- Pain in the lower back or sides

TREATING WITH SELF-CARE

- Drink 8 to 16, 8-ounce glasses of water per day
- Take antibiotics as prescribed and pain relievers as needed

SEE A DOCTOR IF:

- You have a fever, chills, vomiting, and/or nausea
- You also have pain in your lower back
- You pass blood in your urine or it is dark and cloudy
- You have pain in your abdomen or bladder
- It hurts to have sexual intercourse
- The medicine used to clear up the infection causes side effects

PREVENTING URINARY TRACT INFECTION

- Drink 8 to 16, 8-ounce glasses of water per day
- Urinate at the first feeling of need
- Wear cotton underwear to keep dry, and loose clothing to allow skin to breathe
- If you use a diaphragm, keep it clean and checked regularly for proper fitting
- Avoid intercourse until the infection clears

CHAPTER THREE:

Managing Chronic Conditions

In this chapter of Self-Care Essentials, we'll explore conditions that tend to be chronic in nature. Fourteen conditions will be covered in all, and essential information for the maintenance of good health and well-being will be presented.

IMPORTANT TOPICS COVERED

It is important to note that the conditions addressed in this chapter do not make up a complete list. There are literally hundreds of topics that could have been addressed in this chapter. However, the conditions we have chosen to include were selected based on their prevalence and frequency of occurrence.

We trust that you will find the information contained on the following pages to be beneficial in your efforts to live well by managing chronic conditions.

WORDS TO THE WISE

Throughout this book, we've offered many "words to the wise." This one is especially important. In this day and age, many of us are living longer—a great blessing. However, the longer we live, the more likely we are to live with a chronic condition. Whether or not you're a current sufferer, the information contained in this chapter is valuable. In fact, it's critical to a mindset that emphasizes living well with any health condition.

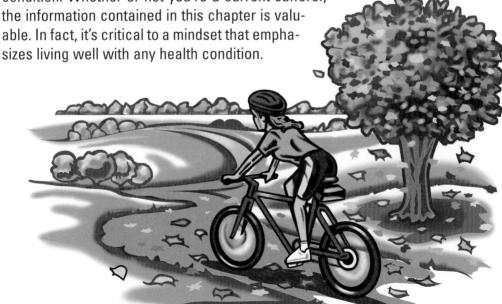

HOW TO TREAT...

Alzheimer's

Alzheimer's disease results in the death of brain cells. This gradual loss of brain cells hinders a person's ability to think clearly. The cause of Alzheimer's disease is not known, but the disease affects about 10% of persons over the age of 65.

SIGNS AND SYMPTOMS

- Gradual memory loss
- A tendency to repeat statements
- The frequent loss of important items
- Confusion
- Tendency to get lost
- Increased irritability, depression, or anxiety
- Gradual loss of personality traits
- Disorientation
- Loss of decision-making skills
- Tendency to wander
- Muscle twitching or convulsions
- Difficulty recognizing friends and family
- Trouble with speech

TREATING WITH SELF-CARE

- **If you suffer**
  - ✓ Fill out an advanced directive to indicate what type of care you wish to receive in various situations should you become unable to communicate your wishes
  - ✓ Get in contact with the Alzheimer's Association

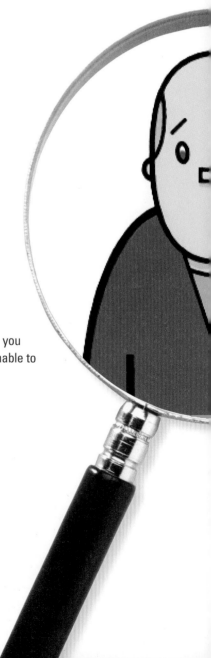

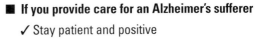

■ **If you provide care for an Alzheimer's sufferer**

✓ Stay patient and positive

✓ Establish and follow a consistent routine

✓ Write out daily activities for the person to keep and follow

✓ Keep things in particular places

✓ Post notes around the home as reminders

✓ Keep the person physically and mentally active

✓ Provide a safe living environment

✓ Research care options, should you become unable to properly provide care

✓ Get help and support

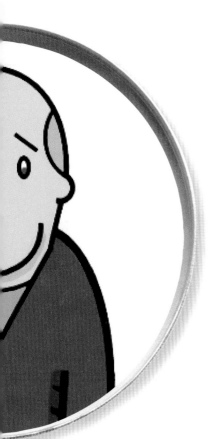

SEE A DOCTOR IF:

■ You begin to show signs and symptoms of Alzheimer's disease

■ A diagnosed person begins to worsen quickly or unexpectedly

■ The person begins to resist care or becomes violent or easily agitated

■ You are providing care for a sufferer and feel you can no longer do so

WORDS TO THE WISE

Most family members that care for an Alzheimer's victim need support themselves. If you know someone that is caring for a sufferer, make sure that you're there for them as well. You can help out by preparing meals, cleaning the house, taking the sufferer for walks or drives, or any number of things.

HOW TO TREAT...

Anemia

Anemia is a condition where the blood's ability to transport oxygen is reduced. There are three primary causes of anemia, including a reduced production of red blood cells, excessive destruction of red blood cells, and excessive blood loss.

SIGNS AND SYMPTOMS

- Fatigue
- Shortness of breath
- Fainting
- Pale skin
- Heavy menstrual flow
- Black, tarry stools

TREATING WITH SELF-CARE

- If you're diagnosed with anemia, visit your doctor and follow the instructions for care
- Eat a well-balanced diet that includes:
  - ✓ Foods high in iron (i.e., green, leafy vegetables, lean red meat, beef, poultry, fish, wheat germ, and iron-fortified cereals)
  - ✓ Foods high in folic acid (i.e., asparagus, brussels sprouts, spinach, romaine lettuce, collard greens, and broccoli)
  - ✓ Raw vegetables
  - ✓ Foods high in vitamin C (i.e., citrus fruits, tomatoes, and strawberries)
- If you drink tea, switch to herbal tea to ensure the proper absorption of nutrients
- Ask a doctor if an iron supplement might be right for you
- Don't smoke and avoid secondhand smoke

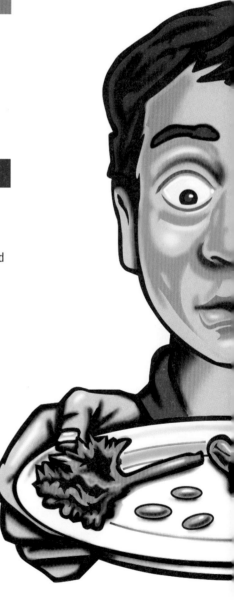

SEE A DOCTOR IF:

■ You experience any symptoms of anemia for no known reason

■ You get dizzy or lightheaded when you stand up or are physically active

■ You have a ringing noise in your ears

■ You are female and experience any of the following:
  ✓ Vaginal bleeding between periods
  ✓ Heavy menstrual bleeding that lasts for several months

WORDS TO THE WISE

In order to prevent anemia, it is important to do two things. First, eat a well-balanced diet. For dietary specifics, refer to the "TREATING WITH SELF-CARE" section on the previous page. Second, get at least 30 minutes of exercise most days of the week. Exercise is always good advice and will help to prevent anemia.

"The first wealth is health."

– RALPH WALDO EMERSON

HOW TO TREAT...

Arthritis

Despite the many kinds of arthritis, these painful conditions all share one thing in common: they involve inflammation or swelling in a joint. There are many different types of arthritis. Consult your doctor for an accurate diagnosis.

SIGNS AND SYMPTOMS

- Joint stiffness
- Joint swelling
- Deep joint pain
- Joint pain during movement and difficulty in movement
- Redness or heat surrounding a joint

TREATING WITH SELF-CARE

- See a doctor on a regular basis and follow the plan of care
- Try heat—a warm shower or bath can do wonders to loosen stiff joints
- Don't spend too much time sitting
- Put each of your joints slowly through its full range of motion 1 to 2 times per day
- Exercise cautiously and regularly with low impact movements such as walking, cycling, and water aerobics
- Get plenty of rest and relax sore, swollen, or tired joints
- Use cold gel packs to relieve pain and reduce swelling
- Take over-the-counter medications for pain relief and inflammation

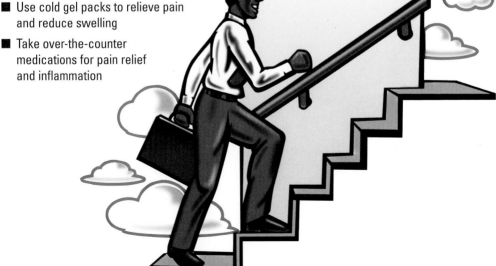

SEE A DOCTOR IF:

- Your joint pain comes with a fever or a skin rash
- The joint is causing intense pain
- Pain, swelling, or redness comes on suddenly
- Pain or swelling is severe and in multiple joints
- The medications prescribed are not effective in controlling the pain or are causing side effects
- Self-care treatment provides little or no relief

PREVENTING ARTHRITIS

- Keep impact on joints low
- Maintain a healthy weight
- Get at least 30 minutes of exercise most days of the week
- Get adequate follow-up treatment for all injuries

"A warm shower or bath can do wonders to loosen stiff joints."

WORDS TO THE WISE

Arthritis is a chronic condition that can cause a great deal of pain and severely limit an individual's activities. If you or someone you know is affected, remember that emotional health is also important. It's important to STAY POSITIVE! There may not be a cure for arthritis, but there are a number of things you can do to lessen the adverse effects of the condition.

HOW TO TREAT...

Cancer

The term cancer refers to a broad range of medical conditions in which cells of the body become abnormal. These cells grow and become harmful or malignant to the individual. Cancer is the second leading cause of death for Americans. In most cases, cancer is treatable if it is detected early enough. The exact causes of cancer are not yet known, but they appear to be linked in large part to dietary and environmental factors.

SIGNS AND SYMPTOMS

- A change in your urination or bowel movement habits
- A lump or thickening detected in the testicle, breast, or anywhere else
- A wound that takes longer than usual to heal
- Significant change in a wart or mole
- Indigestion or difficulty swallowing
- Unusual rectal discharge, vaginal bleeding, or bleeding from any part of the body
- Persistent cough or hoarseness
- Unexplained weight loss

RISK FACTORS

- Significant or routine exposure to the sun, nuclear radiation, x-rays, or radon gas
- Tobacco use and/or excessive use of alcohol
- Polluted air and water
- Certain dietary factors, including too much fat and char-broiled or char-grilled meats
- Exposure to chemicals such as wood dust, asbestos, benzenes, nickel, radioactive materials, and some ingredients in cigarette smoke
- Family history of cancer

TREATING WITH SELF-CARE

- Follow all recommendations of your doctor
- Perform regular self-examinations, such as testicular or breast self-exams, noting any changes, lumps, or thickening—identification is a key part of cancer self-care
- Look your body over frequently and note any significant changes in warts, moles, or wounds that have not healed
- Schedule regular checkups with your doctor for a complete exam

SEE A DOCTOR IF:

- You detect any abnormalities during the course of a self-examination or have any reason to be suspicious of a developing cancer
- You are undergoing cancer treatment and are suffering from unusual side effects

PREVENTING CANCER

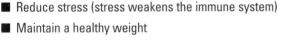

- Keep your dietary fat intake below 30% of your total calories
- Eat plenty of fruits and vegetables, including brussels sprouts, cabbage, and broccoli—these foods contain cancer-fighting chemicals
- Consume alcoholic beverages in moderation
- Don't smoke or use tobacco products and avoid secondhand smoke
- Limit your exposure to the sun and use sunscreen during extended periods of exposure (preferably with an SPF of 15 to 30)
- Avoid the sun altogether during the sun's peak hours (10:00 a.m. to 2:00 p.m.)
- Reduce stress (stress weakens the immune system)
- Maintain a healthy weight

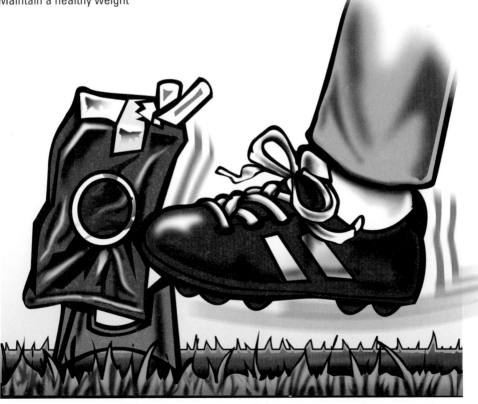

HOW TO TREAT...

Diabetes

Diabetes occurs when the body does not make enough insulin or is unable to adequately use insulin. Insulin is a hormone that helps the body use blood sugar for energy. There are two main types of diabetes—Type I and Type II.

Type I diabetics do not produce enough insulin. This form of diabetes usually develops before the age of 30.

Type II diabetics still produce adequate amounts of insulin, but their bodies are unable to use it effectively. This form of diabetes usually occurs after the age of 40.

SIGNS AND SYMPTOMS

Drowsiness
Itching
A family history of diabetes
Blurred vision
Excessive weight
Tingling, numbness, or pain in the extremities
Easy fatigue
Skin infection, slow healing of cuts and scratches, especially on the feet

Constant urination
Abnormal thirst
Unusual hunger
The rapid loss of weight
Irritability
Obvious weakness and fatigue
Nausea and vomiting

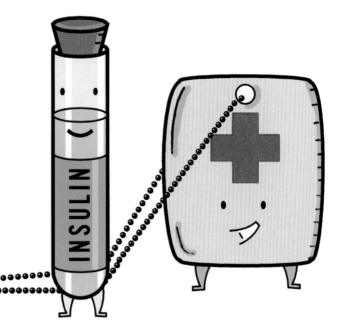

TREATING WITH SELF-CARE

The specific treatments for diabetes depend on the type and severity of the condition. However, the general self-care strategy is the same—maintain normal blood sugar levels. The following tips can help.

- Eat a well-balanced diet that includes:
  - ✓ Proper amounts (as indicated by a doctor) of protein, fat, and carbohydrates
  - ✓ Proper amounts of dietary fiber
  - ✓ Less than 30% of fat in your total daily calories
  - ✓ Limited alcohol consumption
  - ✓ Regular eating intervals
- Get at least 30 minutes of exercise most days of the week
- Maintain a healthy weight
- Take prescribed medications (medications may include oral capsules or tablets and/or insulin injections as prescribed by a doctor)
- Monitor blood sugar levels at home

SEE A DOCTOR IF:

- You notice the above signs and symptoms
- You are diagnosed with diabetes and you experience life-threatening complications
- You are diagnosed with diabetes and you are having difficulty following your self-care regimen
- You are diagnosed with diabetes and are suffering emotional complications because of the condition

WORDS TO THE WISE

Persons living with diabetes can live and enjoy a normal and long life. Establishing a self-care routine with proper support from a doctor is key. As time goes on, many people living with diabetes begin to more fully understand that it is a manageable life condition that doesn't have to affect "quality of life."

HOW TO TREAT...

Emphysema

Emphysema is a chronic lung condition that occurs when the air sacs in the lungs enlarge and lose their elasticity. This reduces the ability of the lungs to take in oxygen. As a result, sufferers are often short of breath and have difficulty performing even the most basic daily tasks. Smoking is the most common cause of the condition, making emphysema a very preventable condition.

SIGNS AND SYMPTOMS

- Wheezing
- Fatigue
- Chronic coughing
- Shortness of breath during simple physical activities

TREATING WITH SELF-CARE

- Follow your doctor's instructions carefully—this includes taking any medications or following other treatments that may have been prescribed
- Don't smoke and avoid secondhand smoke
- Avoid dusty, polluted environments
- Get at least 30 minutes of exercise most days of the week
- Eat a well-balanced diet
- Drink 8 to 16, 8-ounce glasses of water per day
- Perform breathing exercises to improve your breathing ability

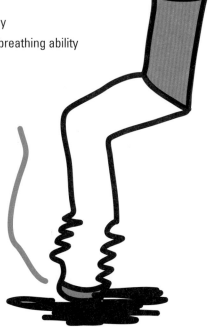

SEE A DOCTOR IF:

■ You are experiencing any of the signs or symptoms for the first time

■ You are having severe symptoms

■ You are interested in learning how you can quit smoking

■ You are concerned that your lifestyle or environment may be putting you at risk for emphysema

PREVENTING EMPHYSEMA

■ Don't smoke and avoid secondhand smoke

■ Limit your exposure to dusty, polluted environments

■ Get at least 30 minutes of exercise most days of the week

■ Eat a well-balanced diet

WORDS TO THE WISE

You may have noticed that the prevention of emphysema is strikingly similar to its treatment. We've listed both the prevention and treatment on these pages to drive home a point. Although emphysema cannot be cured, it can easily be prevented. What's more, its damaging effects can be slowed, and its symptoms eased. If someone you know has emphysema, be supportive of their lifestyle changes and recognize the severity of their condition.

HOW TO TREAT...

Heart Disease

Heart disease, or coronary artery disease, is the leading cause of death in our country. This serious condition is the narrowing or blocking of the coronary arteries, which carry blood to the heart. When an artery is blocked, the flow of blood is cut off, and a heart attack can occur. There are a variety of factors that contribute to heart disease. Here's what you need to know.

SIGNS AND SYMPTOMS

■ **Know the signs of a heart attack:**
- ✓ Persistent pressure or pain in the chest, even if not intense
- ✓ Pressure or pain that spreads to the shoulder, neck, arm, or jaw
- ✓ Nausea or vomiting with chest pain
- ✓ A cold sweat
- ✓ Difficulty breathing and/or swallowing
- ✓ Dizziness/fainting
- ✓ Sense of doom

TREATING WITH SELF-CARE

- ■ Follow your doctor's instructions carefully
- ■ Take all medications precisely as prescribed
- ■ Don't smoke and avoid secondhand smoke
- ■ Lose excess weight if you are overweight
- ■ Eat a well-balanced diet and follow any nutritional instructions from your doctor
- ■ Get at least 30 minutes of exercise most days of the week
- ■ Reduce stress
- ■ Get adequate rest and relaxation

WORDS TO THE WISE

With so many lives taken by heart disease, it is important that you do all you can to prevent the disease. Some of these factors we can control, some of them we cannot. Focus on what you can control and understand your risks.

SEE A DOCTOR IF:

■ You experience any of the mentioned signs and symptoms for the first time

■ You experience severe symptoms

■ You are having a difficult time performing even basic daily tasks

■ You have a family history of heart disease and you have not recently had a medical checkup

PREVENTING HEART DISEASE

■ **Know the facts:**

✓ Find out if your family has a history of heart disease

✓ Have your blood pressure checked regularly and follow your doctor's instructions to keep it from getting too high

✓ Get regular medical checkups and be sure to have your cholesterol checked

■ **Treat your body well:**

✓ Don't smoke and avoid secondhand smoke

✓ Eat a well-balanced diet

✓ Get at least 30 minutes of exercise most days of the week

✓ Reduce stress

✓ Get adequate rest and relaxation

✓ Control diabetes (if diabetic)

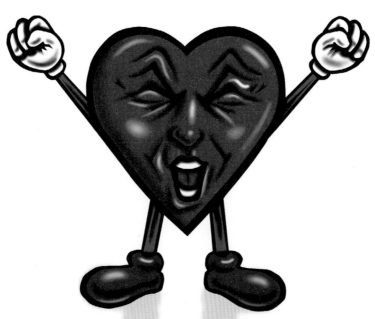

HOW TO TREAT...

Hemorrhoids

Hemorrhoids are swollen blood vessels around the anus and in the rectum. They usually result from repeated pressure in the rectal or anal veins. That pressure can come from straining to pass hard stools, repeated heavy lifting, obesity, pregnancy, childbirth, or other causes. Hemorrhoids can develop either inside or outside of the anus. The good news is that hemorrhoids are a treatable, reversible medical condition.

SIGNS AND SYMPTOMS

- Rectal itching, burning, pain, inflammation, or tenderness, especially during bowel movements
- Rectal bleeding
- Blood on the toilet or toilet tissue
- A lump that can be felt in the anus
- A mucus discharge following a bowel movement

TREATING WITH SELF-CARE

- **Drink, eat, and do**
  - ✓ Drink 8 to 16, 8-ounce glasses of water per day
  - ✓ Eat plenty of high-fiber foods, such as wheat, bran, fresh fruits, and nearly all vegetables
  - ✓ Get at least 30 minutes of exercise most days of the week
- **Treatment and relief**
  - ✓ Take showers or baths every day and thoroughly cleanse the skin around your anus with warm water
  - ✓ Take warm baths without bubbles, oils, or other additives
  - ✓ Apply ice packs to reduce irritation and swelling
  - ✓ Apply over-the-counter medicated creams or other agents to relieve itching and irritation
- **Do the right thing**
  - ✓ Wear cotton underwear and loose clothing to minimize moisture in the anal area
  - ✓ Pass bowel movements as soon as you feel the urge
  - ✓ Don't strain during bowel movements
  - ✓ Lose any excess weight
  - ✓ Try to avoid sitting or standing for long periods of time—take breaks and move around frequently

SEE A DOCTOR IF:

- You experience significant blood loss
- Your hemorrhoids get infected
- Pain from your hemorrhoids lasts longer than 1 week
- You have a hard lump where your hemorrhoids used to be
- You have rectal bleeding that lasts longer than 2 weeks
- Your hemorrhoids are extremely painful or keep you from performing basic daily activities

PREVENTING HEMORRHOIDS

- Drink 8 to 16, 8-ounce glasses of water per day
- Eat a well-balanced diet high in dietary fiber
- Take showers or baths every day
- Avoid straining during bowel movements
- Avoid prolonged sitting during bowel movements
- Pass bowel movements as soon as you feel the urge
- Consider stool softeners if necessary

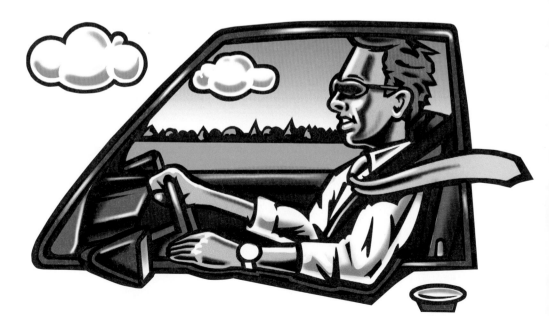

HOW TO TREAT...

Hernias

A hernia occurs when a body part protrudes through the abnormally weakened wall that contains it. The most common hernias are the inguinal and hiatal hernias. Inguinal hernias occur when the lining of the lower abdominal wall weakens and part of the intestine protrudes out. Hiatal hernias occur when the stomach protrudes through the opening in the diaphragm and into the chest cavity.

SIGNS AND SYMPTOMS

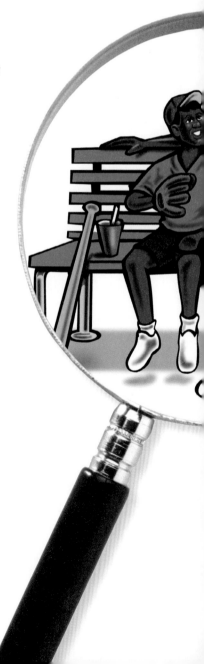

■ **Inguinal Hernias**
- ✓ A gurgling feeling or a sense that something has given way
- ✓ A bulge in the groin or scrotum
- ✓ Pain or discomfort in the groin
- ✓ Abdominal swelling
- ✓ A feeling of pressure or weakness in the abdomen

■ **Hiatal Hernias**
- ✓ Heartburn
- ✓ Belching
- ✓ Hiccuping
- ✓ Chest pain
- ✓ Regurgitation
- ✓ Sour, bitter taste at the back of the throat

TREATING WITH SELF-CARE

■ **Inguinal Hernias**
- ✓ Avoid heavy lifting that causes straining
- ✓ Learn and use appropriate lifting techniques
- ✓ Don't strain during bowel movements
- ✓ Lose excess weight if you are overweight

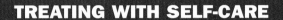
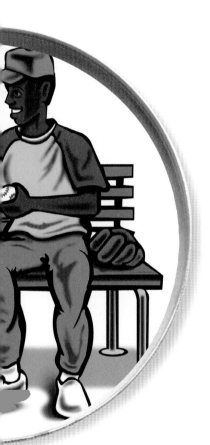

TREATING WITH SELF-CARE

■ **Hiatal Hernias**

- ✓ Avoid irritating foods, such as spicy or highly acidic foods
- ✓ Take antacids to reduce heartburn and indigestion
- ✓ Elevate the head of your bed to keep stomach contents from flowing backward
- ✓ If indigestion occurs after big meals, try eating smaller, more frequent meals
- ✓ Avoid eating 3 hours before bedtime
- ✓ Avoid lying down for 2 hours after eating
- ✓ Avoid foods high in fat—they delay digestion

SEE A DOCTOR IF:

- ■ Your hernia becomes painful or extremely bothersome
- ■ The skin over a hernia becomes red
- ■ Heartburn or indigestion continues for more than 2 weeks despite self-care treatment
- ■ You have severe pain in the groin area combined with nausea, vomiting, and a fever
- ■ You are unable to massage a hernia back into place when lying down

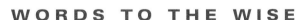

WORDS TO THE WISE

Hernias cannot be prevented or cured through self-care. If you have a hernia and it causes you no discomfort, you do not need to make any drastic lifestyle changes. If you are bothered by the condition, talk to your doctor about possible hernia repairs.

HOW TO TREAT...

High Blood Cholesterol

Cholesterol is a type of fat that is present in every cell of our bodies and is needed for proper cell function. However, excessive amounts of cholesterol (high blood cholesterol) can start to build up as plaque in our arteries, causing them to narrow. When this happens, blood flow is reduced and the chance of a blockage (heart attack) increases.

It is important to note that there are two types of cholesterol, good and bad. Low-density lipoprotein (LDL) is the bad cholesterol that can build up in our arteries. High-density lipoprotein (HDL) is the good cholesterol that helps clear the LDL cholesterol from the arteries.

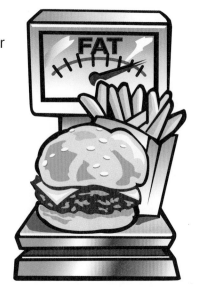

RISK FACTORS

- A family history of high blood cholesterol or heart disease
- Age of 45 or higher for males and 55 or higher for females
- Smoking
- High blood pressure (140/90 mmHg or higher)
- Diabetes
- A diet high in saturated fat
- Physical inactivity

CHOLESTEROL NUMBERS

	TOTAL CHOLESTEROL	HDL (Good) CHOLESTEROL	LDL (Bad) CHOLESTEROL
DESIRABLE	below 200	above 40	below 130
BORDERLINE	200 to 239	keep HDL levels as high as possible	130 to 159
DANGER ZONE	240 or higher	below 40	160 or higher

TREATING WITH SELF-CARE

- Follow your doctor's instructions carefully
- Take medications precisely as prescribed
- Eat a well-balanced diet, lowering your fat intake and increasing your fiber intake
- Get at least 30 minutes of exercise most days of the week
- Don't smoke and avoid secondhand smoke
- Lose any excess weight

SEE A DOCTOR IF:

- You have any or a combination of the risk factors
- You experience any of the following symptoms:
  - ✓ Persistent pressure or pain in the chest
  - ✓ Pressure or pain that spreads to the shoulder, neck, arm, and/or jaw
  - ✓ Nausea or vomiting with chest pain
  - ✓ A cold sweat and/or difficulty breathing
  - ✓ Dizziness and/or a sense of doom

PREVENTING HIGH CHOLESTEROL

- **Do your homework**
  - ✓ Find out if your family has a history of heart disease or high blood cholesterol
  - ✓ Have your blood pressure checked regularly
  - ✓ Get regular medical checkups, and be sure to have your cholesterol checked
- **Do the right thing**
  - ✓ Don't smoke and avoid secondhand smoke
  - ✓ Eat a well-balanced diet, low in saturated fat and high in grains, fruits, and vegetables
  - ✓ Avoid frying foods in fat
  - ✓ Use pure virgin olive oil
  - ✓ Get at least 30 minutes of exercise most days of the week
  - ✓ Reduce stress

HOW TO TREAT...

High Blood Pressure

High blood pressure, also known as hypertension, is a condition where blood is pumped through your arteries at a higher pressure than normal. This puts additional strain on the heart, which increases the risk of a number of unhealthy conditions, including heart disease. Ideal blood pressure is 120/80 mmHg or lower for adults. Readings of 140/90 mmHg or higher indicate high blood pressure.

TREATING WITH SELF-CARE

- Follow your doctor's instructions carefully
- Take all medications precisely as prescribed
- Eat a well-balanced diet, low in salt and fat
- Consume alcohol in moderation, if at all
- Get at least 30 minutes of exercise most days of the week
- Don't smoke and avoid secondhand smoke
- Lose any excess weight
- Reduce stress

SEE A DOCTOR IF:

- Your blood pressure reaches 140/90 mmHg on 2 or more occasions
- You suspect you are suffering side effects from your blood pressure medication
- You have high blood pressure and:
  - ✓ Your blood pressure suddenly rises
  - ✓ Your blood pressure elevates to 180/110 mmHg or higher
- You have a family history of high blood pressure and would like to have a checkup

WORDS TO THE WISE

High blood pressure is one of the most common health conditions in our nation. Frighteningly, many of the people who have the condition don't know they have it, hence its nickname, "the silent killer." This is why it is so important to have your blood pressure regularly checked at a doctor's office, community health center, or fitness center.

PREVENTING HIGH BLOOD PRESSURE

- Find out if your family has a history of heart disease or high blood cholesterol
- Have your blood pressure checked every 4 to 6 months by a medical professional
- Get regular medical checkups and be sure to have your cholesterol checked
- Don't smoke and avoid secondhand smoke
- Maintain a healthy body weight
- Eat a well-balanced diet, lowering your fat intake and increasing your fiber intake
- Get at least 30 minutes of exercise most days of the week
- Get adequate rest and relaxation
- Reduce stress
- Take medication to control your blood pressure and cholesterol levels as directed by your doctor

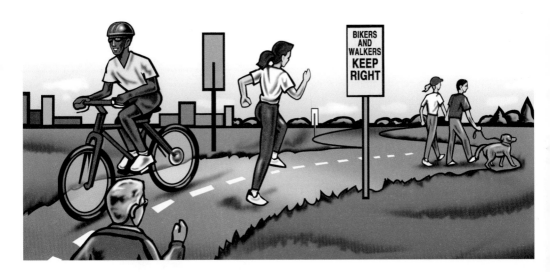

BIKERS AND WALKERS KEEP RIGHT

HOW TO TREAT...

HIV & AIDS

AIDS stands for "acquired immunodeficiency syndrome," and is caused by the human immunodeficiency virus (HIV). HIV is spread when the blood, semen, or vaginal fluids from a person with HIV enters the body of another person. HIV attacks the body's ability to fight off infection and/or disease.

SIGNS AND SYMPTOMS

■ **Any number of symptoms that develop without cause and persist, including:**

✓ Fatigue

✓ Fever and nighttime sweating

✓ Loss of appetite

✓ Weight loss

✓ Diarrhea

✓ Sores in the mouth

✓ Swollen glands in the neck, armpits, or groin

✓ Persistent dry cough

✓ Shortness of breath

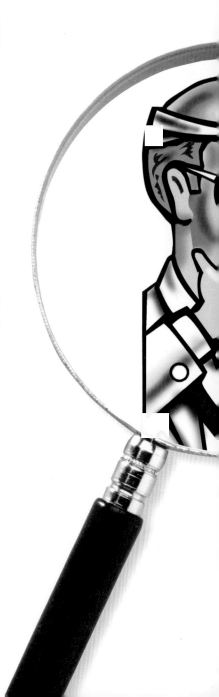

TREATING WITH SELF-CARE

■ **Caring for yourself**

✓ First and foremost, if you have engaged in any behavior that could lead to HIV infection, see a doctor and get tested

✓ If you test positive for HIV, follow the care prescribed by your doctor

✓ If your doctor prescribes medications, take these medications exactly as prescribed

✓ Get adequate rest, eat healthfully, reduce stress, exercise, and avoid smoke and other allergens in order to STAY healthy and avoid illness

✓ See a doctor for any wound or infection

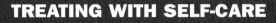

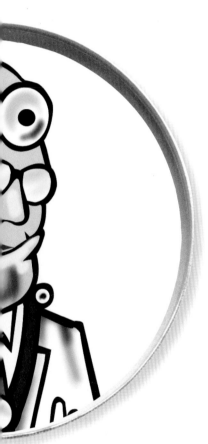

TREATING WITH SELF-CARE

■ **Caring for yourself AND others**

✓ Get emotional support—foster new relationships and strengthen existing ones

✓ If you are in a sexual relationship, make sure your partner gets tested and keep communicating

✓ Stay positive

SEE A DOCTOR IF:

■ Your behavior puts you at risk for getting HIV

■ You have some of the symptoms of HIV listed in this section

■ You have been diagnosed with HIV and:

✓ Come down with an illness

✓ Experience numbness or unexplained pain

✓ Experience personality or psychological changes

✓ Are considering beginning a new sexual relationship

✓ Feel like you can no longer cope with your condition or the stress of life

PREVENTING HIV & AIDS

■ The best prevention is to abstain from sexual contact of any kind until you are in a committed relationship with a person who is HIV negative

■ If you choose to have sexual contact before this time, always use latex protection in all forms of sexual contact (this includes vaginal, anal, and oral sex)—however, this does not guarantee the prevention of infection

■ Don't inject drugs with needles

HOW TO TREAT...

Migraines

Migraines are a specific type of headache caused by the widening or shrinking of blood vessels in your head. These headaches are generally severe and are often recurring. The pain is often described as "piercing" or "throbbing."

SIGNS AND SYMPTOMS

- Pain on one particular side of the head
- Nausea and vomiting
- Flashes of light and/or distorted vision before the headache
- Tingling sensation on the face before the headache
- Ringing ears
- Sensitivity to light and/or sound

TREATING WITH SELF-CARE

- Go to a quiet, dark place and lie down at the first sign of a migraine
- Take medication as prescribed by a doctor (some medications will work better than others—don't hesitate to ask your doctor to try a different medication if needed)
- Apply a cold pack or a cool, moist cloth to your forehead
- Gently massage your neck and shoulders
- Breathe slowly and deeply
- Try to relax
- Always keep a record or log of your headaches so you can precisely note any changes

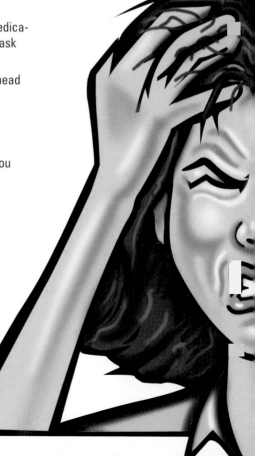

SEE A DOCTOR IF:

- You suspect your headaches are migraines
- Your migraines seem to be getting worse or more frequent
- A headache is accompanied by any of the following:
  - ✓ Weakness
  - ✓ Paralysis
  - ✓ Numbness
  - ✓ Visual disturbances
  - ✓ Slurred speech
  - ✓ Confusion
  - ✓ Fever
- Your headache is like none you've ever had before
- A headache strikes suddenly and severely

PREVENTING MIGRAINES

- Keep track of your headaches, noting events or situations that seem to trigger migraines—alter your lifestyle to avoid these triggers
- Reduce stress—do what you can to loosen up and have fun
- Get at least 30 minutes of exercise most days of the week, but never exercise during a migraine attack

HOW TO TREAT...

Sleep Apnea

Sleep apnea is a condition in which the sufferer stops breathing for short periods of time during a night's sleep. People with this condition often snore and awake with a quick jerk or gasp. It is usually caused by a blockage in the upper airway.

SIGNS AND SYMPTOMS

- Snoring
- Awaking with a jerk or gasp
- Sleepiness or fatigue throughout the day
- Irritability
- Lack of concentration
- Dozing off while driving or working
- Morning headache

TREATING WITH SELF-CARE

- First of all, if you suspect sleep apnea, see a doctor immediately—they may be able to fit you with a device to safeguard your health
- Take any prescribed medications as recommended—these may include nasal decongestants
- Lose weight—research indicates a link between excess weight and sleep apnea
- Try sleeping on your stomach or side
- Avoid alcohol, caffeine, and tobacco before going to bed
- Establish a sleep routine

SEE A DOCTOR IF:

- You have not been diagnosed with sleep apnea and suspect that you may be a sufferer
- You have indications that your condition is worsening
- The medications and self-care treatments do not produce relief from the symptoms
- Your fatigue during the day is preventing you from doing your work effectively
- You suspect medications are causing or worsening the condition

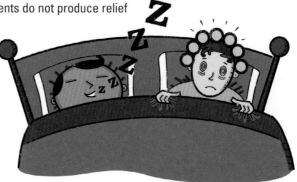

CHAPTER FOUR:

Taking Medications

Taking medications, prescribed or over-the-counter (OTC), is serious business. Failure to follow directions can be very dangerous, even life-threatening. But, medications can also improve health and well-being. In this chapter, we'll provide valuable information and practical tips for getting the most out of medications.

5 ESSENTIALS FOR TAKING MEDICATIONS

1. Understand what medications can do

In this first section of the chapter, we'll provide the information necessary to approach medications with the caution and optimism they deserve.

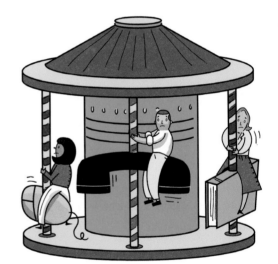

2. Take responsibility for the medications you take

With the information presented in this section, you'll be able to confidently take your medications with accuracy and safety.

3. Cut the cost of your medications

Let's face it, medications are expensive. There are, however, things we can do to save money. Here, we'll give advice for saving big on these little wonders.

4. Keep medication records

To help ensure that medications are taken accurately and in a timely manner, we'll give you some tips and tools for writing down medication information.

5. Know how to use over-the-counter medications

Over-the-counter medications play a big role in our lives and health. Understanding how to use them safely and effectively is a key aspect in personal health.

STEP 1...

Understand What Medications Can Do

Part of the "how to" when it comes to medications is maximizing the benefits and minimizing any unwanted side effects. Unfortunately, most of us just hope for the best. It's time to quit hoping. Here's some of what medications can do.

ACCENTUATE THE POSITIVE

■ **Medications can relieve pains such as:**
- ✓ Headaches
- ✓ Backaches
- ✓ Earaches

■ **Medications can fight infections such as:**
- ✓ Infected wounds
- ✓ Strep throat

■ **Medications can reduce inflammations such as:**
- ✓ Arthritic inflammation
- ✓ Inflammation from injuries
- ✓ Inflammation from sinusitis

■ **Medications can treat digestive disorders such as:**
- ✓ Upset stomach
- ✓ Diarrhea
- ✓ Constipation
- ✓ Nausea and vomiting

AND SO MUCH MORE

The list above merely scratches the surface, but it does make one thing perfectly clear— medications play a significant role in our lives. All too often we take medications for granted. And while we shouldn't lean on them for every minor health issue, we should appreciate them for what they can do and use them wisely.

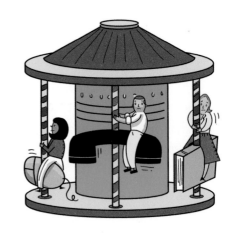

ELIMINATE THE NEGATIVE

Negative or adverse reactions can occur as a result of medication use and misuse very easily. But with the right information we can better protect ourselves and identify problems as soon as they arise.

COMMON PROBLEMS WITH MEDICATIONS

- Chemical addiction
- Allergic reactions
- Side effects
- Drug-drug interactions
- Food-drug interactions
- Overmedication
- Addiction and dependence

ADVERSE REACTIONS

- **Physical problems include:**
  - ✓ Nausea, vomiting and/or dehydration
  - ✓ Indigestion, constipation, diarrhea and/or problems with urination
  - ✓ Bruises and/or skin rashes
  - ✓ Dizziness, confusion, loss of balance and/or disorientation
  - ✓ Blurred or double vision
  - ✓ Insomnia
  - ✓ Fast or uneven heartbeat
  - ✓ Difficulty breathing
- **Psychological problems include:**
  - ✓ Irritability
  - ✓ Depression
  - ✓ Nervousness
  - ✓ Uneasiness
  - ✓ Forgetfulness

Medications need to be approached as powerful tools that should be used with cautious optimism. With this responsible approach, we can accentuate the positive side of medications and eliminate the negative side (or at least come close). The next section will give you some tips on how to do just that—take responsibility.

STEP 2...

Take Responsibility

Responsibility with your doctor or pharmacist

When receiving a prescription or over-the-counter medication, don't be afraid to ask questions. Here are some questions you'll want to ask.

■ Should the drug be taken with water, with food, on an empty stomach, in the morning or evening?

■ How much of the drug should be taken each time, and how frequently?

■ What should be done if a dose is missed?

■ Are there side effects?

■ Are there any food or drug interactions to be aware of?

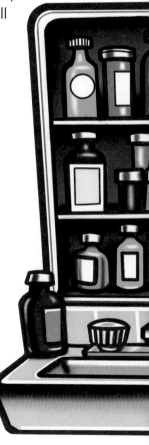

Responsibility on your own

It's up to the consumer to take medications accurately. Try the following tips to make things a bit easier.

■ Set an alarm to remind you to take medications (a digital wristwatch may be helpful)

■ Coordinate medications with another daily occurrence (breakfast, lunch, or dinner are the most common)

■ Mark your calendar as a reminder to get refills

■ Discard old medications to avoid confusion (contact your pharmacist for proper drug disposal recommendations in your area)

■ Try a pillbox to help you keep track of what medications to take at what times

■ Never share medications with anyone, and never take someone else's medications

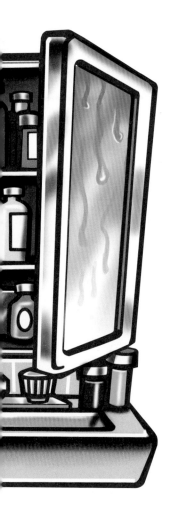

Responsibility at home

Try these tips for raising your level of responsibility at home.

- Keep doctor, pharmacist, and emergency phone numbers handy
- Organize your medicine cabinet
- Finish all medications
- Try to make taking your medication a habit, like brushing your teeth
- Make sure all medications are child-proof
- If you experience side effects, keep a written record of them

Responsibility away from home

Here are some things you may want to consider when you're out and about.

- Pick a pharmacy and stick with it to ensure that all prescription records are on file at one place
- Let your pharmacist know what your ailments are and all the medications you take to treat them
- Write important medical information on a card and keep it in your wallet or handbag
- Always wear important drug allergy bracelets
- Be sure you inform your doctor or pharmacist of any/all specific medical conditions

WORDS TO THE WISE

One final point cannot be overlooked. Contrary to popular belief, medications should never be kept in the medicine cabinet. Heat and steam from showers and baths can cause some drugs to deteriorate rapidly, which can lead to harmful side effects. Medicines should be stored in cool, dark, and dry places, such as the top shelf of a closet. And preferably, all your medications should be kept in a lockbox.

STEP 3...

Cut Medication Costs

People have a lot to say when it comes to medications—not the least of which is their expense. Even over-the-counter medications can be a real hit to the pocketbook. There are some things that can help save some money without putting you in medical jeopardy.

SAVE MONEY:

■ **Talk to a professional**

✓ Tell a doctor you have financial concerns about your medications

✓ Talk to a doctor about ideas on how to save money on medications

✓ Tell a doctor you would like samples of the medication (sometimes you'll be able to get a limited amount of the drug for little or no cost)

✓ Ask about generic equivalents

✓ Ask for a senior citizen's discount, if applicable

✓ Check with your insurance provider about medication coverage

■ **Be resourceful**

✓ Keep your eyes open for sales on over-the-counter medications

✓ Buy in bulk—if you will need to take a specific medication for an extended period of time, ask about getting a large amount for a reduced rate

✓ Check prices at a variety of pharmacies

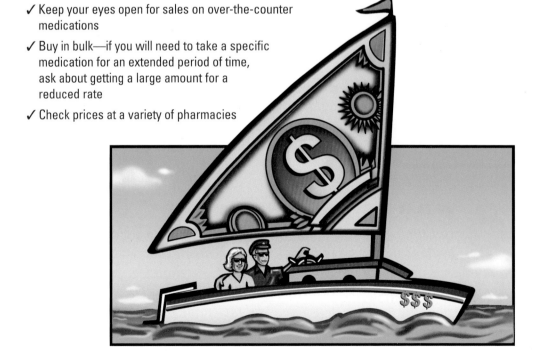

STEP 4...

Keep Medication Records

So far, the material presented in this section has offered valuable information for understanding medications and has also presented several tips for taking medications responsibly. But, another important aspect still needs to be addressed—the documentation of your medications.

As we've seen, medications are powerful tools that need to be treated with cautious optimism. We just can't take medications in a casual manner and hope for the best.

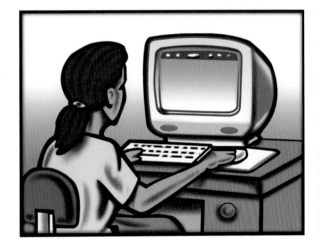

So how do we stop hoping and start anticipating positive improvements to our health and well-being? The answer is twofold. First, we must know the facts presented in the previous pages inside and out. And second, we've got to keep written records of the medications we take and how we take them.

On the following pages, we'll give you some helpful guidelines for creating written medication records.

Continued on next page...

STEP 4...

Keep Medication Records

DETAILED MEDICATION RECORD

The first step in documenting your medications is to chart out the specific information on all the medications that you take. You can use the chart on these pages to help determine your medication specifics and recall them with just a glance. Simply list all the medications you take in the spaces provided and fill in the remaining information.

	Medication Name	Purpose	Color & Shape	Expiration Date
1)				
2)				
3)				
4)				
5)				
6)				
7)				

List all medications you take in the spaces provided.

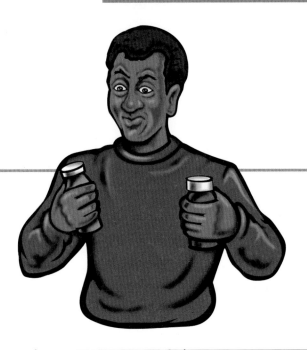

With or Without Food	When and How Much to Take	Doctor's Name/Phone	Side Effects

WORDS TO THE WISE

It's important to do everything possible to stay on a medication schedule. Add to this chart if necessary and remember to keep it updated. Your medication record is the key to getting the maximum benefit and minimum amount of side effects from your medications.

Continued on next page…

STEP 4...

Keep Medication Records

GENERAL MEDICATION CARD

The general medication card and instructions in this section are a supplement to the detailed medication record presented on the previous pages. This general medication card is the next step in documenting your medications and should be carried with you at all times. Here's what you'll want to do.

- Fill out the medication card in this section based on the information from your detailed medication record
- Keep your medication card up-to-date (updating your record should be done twice a year or when any important information changes)
- Keep your medication card with you at all times (keep all of this information on a business-sized card and carry it with you)
- Always be sure to bring your medication card with you when you visit your physician or pharmacist

Here is the information you'll want to include on your medication card:

Front of Card

NAME: _____

PRIMARY DOCTOR: _____

TELEPHONE NUMBER: _____

PHARMACY: _____

TELEPHONE NUMBER: _____

DRUG ALLERGIES: _____

OTHER INFORMATION: _____

Back of Card

I take the following medications/vitamins every day:

_____
_____
_____

I take the following medications/vitamins occasionally or as needed:

_____
_____
_____

YOU may know which medications you're currently taking, but in the case of an emergency, this card might be the only immediate resource available for someone who comes to your aid.

STEP 5...

Know How to Use OTC Medications

Over-the-counter (OTC) medications can be quite effective in treating a wide variety of conditions. But, OTC medications still require a great deal of responsibility and caution. Consider the following information.

USING OTC MEDICATIONS EFFECTIVELY

■ **Protect yourself**

- ✓ Read the directions carefully
- ✓ Research the active ingredients
- ✓ Take only the recommended daily amount
- ✓ Check to see if the protective seals are intact
- ✓ Ensure that the expiration date has not been exceeded
- ✓ Check for interaction warnings

■ **Protect your family**

- ✓ Keep all medications (prescription and non-prescription) out of the reach of children
- ✓ Follow age recommendations found on the label
- ✓ Never increase the dose for an extremely sick child
- ✓ Know the correct amount abbreviations (TBSP = tablespoon and TSP = teaspoon)
- ✓ Always supervise young children
- ✓ Explain to your children that taking medications must be done with an adult

Continued on next page...

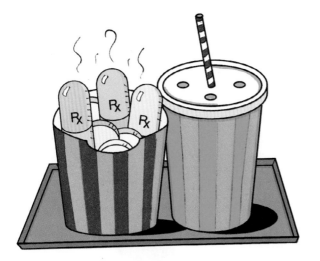

STEP 5...

Know How to Use OTC Medications

Know what to keep on hand

- General pain relievers (aspirin, acetaminophen, ibuprofen)
- Cough syrup
- Antacids
- Antihistamines
- Decongestants
- Eye drops
- Triple antibiotic ointment (Neosporin)
- Aloe vera rub
- Activated charcoal and syrup of ipecac (for poisonings)

Know what to use and when

- **Use general pain relievers for:**
  - ✓ Fevers
  - ✓ General aches and pains
  - ✓ Headache
- **Use antacids for:**
  - ✓ Indigestion
  - ✓ Heartburn
  - ✓ Digestive discomfort

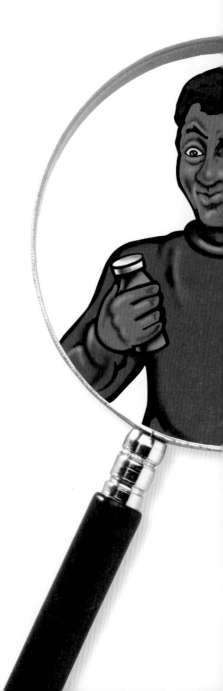

Always read the directions carefully when taking any kind of medication.

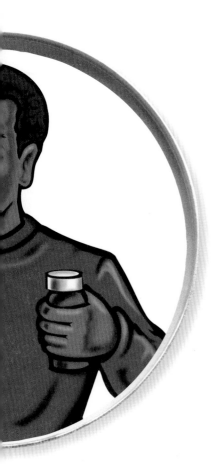

■ **Use antihistamines for:**
- ✓ Relief of allergy symptoms
- ✓ The clearing of sinuses

■ **Use triple antibiotic ointment for:**
- ✓ Infections
- ✓ Scrapes, cuts, and punctures
- ✓ Piercings

■ **Use aloe vera rub for:**
- ✓ Burns
- ✓ Sunburns
- ✓ Scrapes, cuts, and punctures

WORDS TO THE WISE

If they are used effectively, over-the-counter medications can be one of the most powerful weapons in your self-care arsenal. This is true of prescription medications as well.

Consider how you currently use medications. Do you need to adjust any of your habits? Is your family using them correctly and safely? If ANY of the information presented in this chapter suggests that a change is in order, we encourage you to do what's good for your health—make the change.

Glossary

A

AIDS: (acquired immune deficiency syndrome) A disease caused by the HIV virus that adversely affects the body's immune system.

ACETAMINOPHEN: A common over-the-counter drug used to reduce pain and fever.

ACNE: An inflammatory condition of the skin in which oils and bacteria build up under the skin and appear as white, black, or red bumps. The condition is most common on the face and upper back.

ACTIVATED CHARCOAL: A substance commonly used to treat poisonings that acts as an absorbent.

ACUTE CONDITION: A condition characterized by its short duration.

ADDICTION: A habitual dependence on a particular substance that may be either physiologically or psychologically based.

ADVANCED DIRECTIVE: A legal document whereby an individual's desired medical care is specifically requested, should they become unable to communicate these wishes at a later time.

ALLERGIC REACTION: An abnormal physiological reaction to a substance.

ALZHEIMER'S DISEASE: A disease with an unknown cause that results in the death of brain cells and reduces the sufferer's ability to think clearly.

ANEMIA: A condition in which oxygen is not adequately circulated throughout the body's blood stream. Most commonly due to a lack of iron or folic acid.

ANGINA: (pectoris) Severe chest pain often radiating from the heart that is associated with a lack of blood flow to the heart.

ANTACID: An agent that counteracts acids in the digestive tract.

ANTIBIOTIC: A chemical substance designed to treat bacterial infections.

ANTI-DIURETIC: A substance that reduces the output of urine.

ANTIHISTAMINE: A drug having an action antagonistic to that of histamine, a powerful stimulant of gastric secretion and constrictor of bronchial muscles.

ANXIETY: A painful uneasiness of mind grounded in anticipation, apprehension, or dread.

ARTHRITIS: Inflammation of one or more joints.

ASPIRIN: An over-the-counter medication used to treat pain, fever, and inflammation.

ASTHMA: An often-allergic respiratory disease in which there is a narrowing of the airways.

ATHLETE'S FOOT: A highly contagious fungal condition affecting the skin, especially the feet.

B

BACKACHE: A general pain in the back caused by a large variety of possible problems.

BLOOD CHOLESTEROL: A type of fat found in cells that is of two types: 1) low-density lipoprotein and 2) high-density lipoprotein.

BLOOD PRESSURE: The measurable pressure of blood against arterial walls. Also a key indicator of cardiovascular health.

BREASTBONE: The sternum or front midline of the rib cage.

BRONCHITIS: Chronic or acute inflammation and constriction of the air passages in the lungs.

BURN: A general term used in this book to denote all three degrees of damage (i.e., first, second, and third) done to the skin by heat or chemicals.

FIRST-DEGREE BURN: A burn affecting only the outer layer of skin (epidermis) and generally treatable as a minor burn with self-care remedies. The skin will be dry and painful to the touch.

SECOND-DEGREE BURN: A burn involving multiple layers of skin. The burned area typically becomes blistered and swollen and may weep.

THIRD-DEGREE BURN: A burn involving all layers of the skin and likely damaging underlying tissue and/or organs. The skin is often charred black or will have a dry, white appearance.

C

CANCER: Any of a variety of malignant tumors.

CARBON MONOXIDE: A colorless, odorless toxic gas.

CHEMICAL ADDICTION: A physiological dependence on a particular substance.

CHEST MUSCLE PAIN: Pain in the chest muscles most commonly caused by strains and bruises.

CHOKING: A stoppage of breathing caused by an obstruction in the airway.

CHRONIC CONDITION: Any number of medical conditions with a long or repetitive nature.

COLD: A viral condition of the respiratory system.

CONSTIPATION: Difficult or infrequent passage of stools.

CORONARY ARTERY DISEASE: The leading cause of death in the United States at the turn of the millennium caused by the clogging of the heart's arteries.

COUGH: A forceful ejection of air from the lungs.

CUT: A slice of the skin typically referred to as a laceration.

Glossary

D

DECONGESTANT: An agent that reduces congestion, primarily used to treat mucus congestion.

DEHYDRATION: The depletion of body fluids.

DIABETES: A condition related to the body's inability to properly metabolize sugar for energy.

> Type I (insulin-dependent) diabetics do not produce enough insulin. This form of diabetes usually develops before the age of 30.

> Type II (non-insulin-dependent) diabetics still produce adequate amounts of insulin, but their bodies are unable to use it effectively. This form of diabetes usually occurs after the age of 40.

DIAGNOSIS: Determination of the identification or classification of a disease.

DIARRHEA: Loose and abnormally frequent passage of stools.

DROWNING: Suffocation in any amount and type of liquid.

DRUG ALLERGY: An unintended and undesired physiological reaction to a medication.

DRUG-DRUG INTERACTION: An unintended and undesired physiological reaction between two or more medications.

E

EARACHE: Pain in the ear associated with any number of various causes.

ECZEMA: An acute or chronic inflammatory condition of the skin characterized by an itchy, red, raised rash on the face, scalp, neck, bend of the elbows and knees, buttocks, thighs, or torso. Blister-like, crusty scales on these areas with possible weeping may also occur.

EMERGENCY CONDITION: A condition in which immediate care is needed.

ESSENTIAL FIRST AID EQUIPMENT: All medical paraphernalia that should be kept on hand and available in a first aid kit.

F

FLU: (influenza) An infectious viral condition that affects the respiratory system and is often associated with a fever, muscle aches, and chills.

FOLIC ACID: A vitamin of the B complex commonly used to treat or prevent nutritional anemia.

FOOD-DRUG INTERACTION: An unintended and undesired physiological reaction between food and a medication.

G

GENERIC EQUIVALENT: The bio-equivalent of a medication developed without the name brand and often sold at a reduced cost.

H

HAY FEVER: A severe, acute allergic reaction in the upper respiratory system and eyes.

HEAD INJURY: An injury to the head caused by some form of impact.

HEADACHE: A pain occurring in the head, typically towards the front or top, but not necessarily confined to those areas.

HEART ATTACK: (myocardial infarction) An interruption to the normal functioning of the heart and its ability to circulate blood throughout the body.

HEART DISEASE: A variety of conditions adversely affecting the heart and circulatory system often culminating in a heart attack.

HEARTBURN: A painful condition in the stomach and esophagus caused by a backflow of excess acid.

HEAT EXHAUSTION: A reaction to excessive heat characterized by nausea, dizziness, sweating, and general weakness.

HEATSTROKE: A reaction to excessive heat characterized by discontinued sweating and a very high body temperature.

HEIMLICH MANEUVER: A technique used to dislodge an object from the airway of a choking victim in which the person providing aid delivers forceful abdominal thrusts from behind the victim.

HEMORRHOID: A painful mass and swelling of veins in the rectum and/or anus.

HERNIA: A protrusion of a body part through a weakened body tissue, typically in the lower abdominal area.

HIATAL HERNIA: A hernia in which part of the stomach protrudes through the esophageal hiatus of the diaphragm.

HIGH BLOOD CHOLESTEROL: A high level of cholesterol in the bloodstream that results in a build-up of plaque on the arterial walls.

HIGH BLOOD PRESSURE: A condition where blood is pumped through the arteries at a higher pressure than normal, putting additional strain on the heart.

HIGH-DENSITY LIPOPROTEIN: (HDL) "Good" cholesterol that is protein-rich and low in fat, correlated with a reduced risk for coronary artery disease.

HIV: (human immunodeficiency virus) A virus spread when the blood, semen, or vaginal fluids from a person with HIV enter the body of another person. HIV attacks the body's ability to fight off infection.

Glossary

I

IBUPROFEN: An over-the-counter medication used to relieve pain and reduce fever and inflammation.

IMMUNE SYSTEM: The system of the body that protects against foreign substances by producing an appropriate protective response.

INDIGESTION: Discomfort and/or difficulty in digesting foods.

INFECTION: Multiplication of undesired bacteria within the body.

INFLAMMATION: A response to injury or physiological abnormality characterized by swelling, redness, and/or inhibited function.

INFLUENZA: (flu) An infectious viral condition that affects the respiratory system and is often associated with a fever, muscle aches, and chills.

INGUINAL HERNIA: A hernia in which the lining of the lower abdominal wall ruptures and part of the intestine balloons out.

INSOMNIA: A prolonged and abnormal inability to sleep.

INSULIN: A hormone produced in the pancreas essential for the metabolism of carbohydrates and in the treatment of diabetes mellitus.

L

LAXATIVE: An agent used to loosen the bowels and relieve constipation.

LOW-DENSITY LIPOPROTEIN: (LDL) "Bad" cholesterol that is protein-poor and high in fat, correlated with an increased risk for coronary artery disease.

M

MENSTRUATION: A discharging of blood and tissue debris from the uterus occurring in females of reproductive age at approximately monthly intervals.

MIGRAINE: A severe recurring headache often accompanied by vision disorders and nausea.

MYOCARDIAL INFARCTION: (heart attack) An interruption to the normal functioning of the heart and its ability to circulate blood throughout the body.

MUCUS: A slippery secretion that is produced by membranes and serves to moisten and protect.

N

NAUSEA: A stomach irritation characterized by an urge to vomit.

NUTRITION: The dietary consumption of all nutrients by an individual.

O

OBESITY: A condition of excess fat tissue carried by an individual.

OVER-THE-COUNTER: (OTC) A medication available without a prescription from a doctor.

OVULATION: The release of a mature ovum (egg) from the ovary.

P

PEAK FLOW METER: A device used to measure the functional volume of the lungs.

PHYSICAL ACTIVITY: Bodily movement that is produced to burn energy and benefit the body.

POISONING: The ingestion of a substance that causes illness, injury, or death.

PULMONARY EMBOLISM: The obstruction of a blood vessel in the lungs.

PUNCTURE: A wound caused by the penetration or stabbing of an object into the skin.

R

RESCUE BREATHING: A procedure used to deliver oxygen to the lungs of a person that is not breathing.

S

SCRAPE: Damage to the surface of the skin, typically referred to as an abrasion.

SEIZURE: Impairment of normal brain functions, causing the cells of the brain to behave in abnormal ways.

SELF-CARE: The process by which an individual is provided with medical information and the means for managing and caring for many aspects of their health independently.

SHOCK: A state of marked physical and mental depression resulting from severe physical injury.

SICKLE CELL ANEMIA: A form of anemia in which cells are C-shaped or crescent-shaped, hindering the ability of the cells to carry oxygen in the blood.

SIDE EFFECT: An effect additional to the desired or intended effect of a drug or other form of therapy, usually undesirable.

SINUS HEADACHES: This rare type of headache is caused by a blockage in the sinus cavity.

SINUSITIS: Inflammation of the lining of one or more of the sinus cavities.

SLEEP APNEA: A temporary stoppage of breathing during sleep.

SORE THROAT: A dryness or irritation in the esophagus.

Glossary

SPRAIN: An injury to a ligament surrounding a joint, but without dislocation.

STING: A puncturing of the skin by an insect.

STRAIN: An injury to a muscle resulting from improper use or overuse.

STREP THROAT: An inflammatory sore throat marked by fever and caused by the streptococci virus.

STRESS: Emotional strain or pressure.

SYRUP OF IPECAC: A substance ingested for the purpose of inducing vomiting in a victim who has been poisoned.

T

TENSION HEADACHE: A common headache associated with anxiety, tension, and the contraction of scalp muscles.

THERMOMETERS: A device used to measure the body temperature of an individual.

TOOTHACHE: A general pain caused by a variety of ailments to the gums and/or teeth.

U

UNCONSCIOUSNESS: A state in which an individual is unresponsive to stimuli. The individual may have also stopped breathing and their heart may have also stopped beating.

V

VITAL SIGNS: Indicators of life in an individual such as pulse rate, breathing rate, blood pressure, and temperature.

VOMITING: The forceful expulsion of matter from the stomach through the mouth.

W

WELL-BEING: The state of being happy and healthy.

Index

Index

Notes

Emergency #'s